Multisystem Inflammatory Syndrome - Natural History

Edited by Nicolás Padilla-Raygoza

Published in London, United Kingdom

Multisystem Inflammatory Syndrome - Natural History
http://dx.doi.org/10.5772/intechopen.111142
Edited by Nicolás Padilla-Raygoza

Contributors
Nicolás Padilla-Raygoza, Faina Linkov, Gilberto Flores-Vargas, María de Jesús Gallardo-Luna, Efraín Navarro-Olivos, Francisco Javier Magos-Vázquez, Cuauhtémoc Sandoval Salazar, Paola Trinidad Villalobos Gútierrez, Oscar Gútierrez Coronado, Vicente Beltrán Campos, Ciprian Ioan Roi, Alexandra Roi, Mircea Riviș, Luz-Ma.-Adriana Balderas-Peña, Daniel Sat-Muñoz, Mario-Alberto Mireles-Ramírez, Brenda-Eugenia Martínez-Herrera, Arnulfo-Hernán Nava-Zavala, Luz-María Cervantes-González, Michelle-Guadalupe Muñoz-García, Benjamín Rubio-Jurado, Mario Salazar Páramo, Eduardo Gómez Sánchez, Carlos-M Nuño-Guzmán, Víctor Manuel Gutiérrez-Gómez, Beatriz Archundia-Jiménez, Rodrigo Miguel González-Sánchez, Jerónimo Amado López-Arriaga, Beatriz X. Pasco-Velázquez, Alejandra Gómez-Flores, Alije Keka-Sylaj

First published in London, United Kingdom, 2024 by IntechOpen
IntechOpen is the global imprint of INTECHOPEN LIMITED, registered in England and Wales, registration number: 11086078, 5 Princes Gate Court, London, SW7 2QJ, United Kingdom

British Library Cataloguing-in-Publication Data
A catalogue record for this book is available from the British Library

Additional hard and PDF copies can be obtained from orders@intechopen.com

Multisystem Inflammatory Syndrome - Natural History
Edited by Nicolás Padilla-Raygoza
p. cm.
Print ISBN 978-0-85466-305-7
Online ISBN 978-0-85466-304-0
eBook (PDF) ISBN 978-0-85466-306-4

For EU product safety concerns:
IN TECH d.o.o., Prolaz Marije Krucifikse Kozulić 3, 51000 Rijeka, Croatia,
info@intechopen.com or visit our website at intechopen.com.

Meet the editor

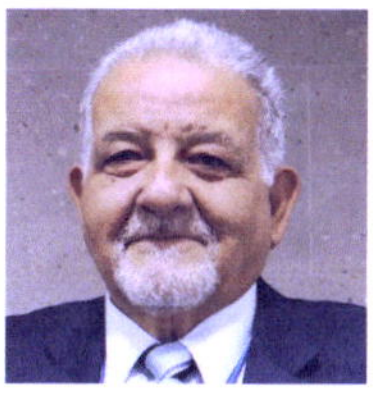

Dr. Nicolás Padilla-Raygoza was a Professor Titular B, Department of Nursing and Obstetrics, Division of Health Sciences and Engineering, Campus Celaya-Salvatierra, University of Guanajuato, Mexico, and Coordinator of Research and Continuous Education, School of Medicine, University of Celaya, México. He is currently a coordinator of research projects at the Institute of Public Health, Guanajuato State. He obtained an MD from Universidad Autónoma de Guadalajara School of Medicine, National Autonomous University of Mexico (UAG-UNAM) in 1984, specialization in pediatrics from the Mexican Council of Certification in 1986, a postgraduate degree in Epidemiology from the University of London in 2001, a master's degree and doctorate in Science from Atlantic International University (AIU) in 2006, and a master's degree in Social Gerontology from the International Iberoamerican University (UNINI Mexico) in 2017. Dr. Padilla-Raygoza has 172 journal articles and 518 book chapters to his credit. He has also edited five books on health. He was recognized as a state researcher on health by the Institute of Public Health, Guanajuato State in 2015, and as a researcher with social impact by the Urbanizadora del Bajío, S.A. (UBSA) in 2016. He was previously a member of the National Researchers System and is a current member of the National System of Researchers from the National Council of Sciences, Humanities, and Technology, and the Mexican Academy of Pediatrics. He is also a fellow of the Royal Society of Public Health.

Contents

Preface

With the emergence of an unknown cause of pneumonia in Wuhan, China, and the subsequent identification and definition of coronavirus disease (COVID-19), the world faced important challenges due to the rapid dissemination of the virus and disease. In May 2020, Mexico reported a case rate of 9.8% [1–3]. As of July 16, 2023, there were 768,037,878 confirmed cases of SARS-COV-2 infection and 6,951,896 deaths due to COVID-19 worldwide. The fatality rate is 0.91%, with COVID affecting 273 countries, territories, and areas [4].

Multisystem inflammatory syndrome (MIS) was initially reported in children in the United Kingdom in April 2020, when an increase in critically ill children with hyperinflammatory shock and evidence of SARS-CoV-2 Infection was described [5]. The United States Centers for Disease Control and Prevention (CDC) and the World Health Organization (WHO) developed definitions for this entity [6–8].

This book provides a comprehensive overview of MIS from the point of view of the natural history of the disease because it is a more didactic way to study the evolution of the syndrome. The book is organized into three sections: an introduction; a discussion of the prepathogenic period, including the ecological triad, before the disease is clinically manifested; and an examination of the clinical stage, which reviews the clinical manifestations, complications, sequelae, and causes of death of MIS.

I want to thank all the authors for their hard work in the elaboration of the chapters. I would also like to thank Publishing Process Manager Laura Divic at IntechOpen for her excellent work and support throughout the publication process.

Dr. Nicolás Padilla-Raygoza
Department of Research and Technological Development,
Directorate of Teaching and Research,
Institute of Public Health from Guanajuato State,
Mexico

References

[1] World Health Organization. Rolling updates on coronavirus disease (COVID-19). Update 23 March 2020. 2020. Available from: https://www.who.int/emergencies/diseases/novel-coronavirus-2019/events-as-they-happen

[2] Carlos WG, De la Cruz C, Cao B, Pasnick S, Jamil S. Novel Wuhan (2019-CoV) coronavirus. American Journal of Respiratory and Critical Care Medicine. 2020;**201**(4):7-8. DOI: 10.1164/rccm.2014P7

[3] Padilla-Raygoza N, Sandoval-Salazar C, Navarro-Olivos E, Gallardo-Luna MJ, Magos-Vázquez FJ, Díaz-Martínez DA. Description of confirmed cases and deaths from COVID-19 in México, until May 6, 2020: An ecological study. Biomedical & Pharmacology Journal. 2020;**13**(3):1471-1476. DOI: 10.13005/bpj/2019

[4] Dirección General de Epidemiología. Coronavirus COVID19 Informe Técnico Semanal. 2 Aug 2023. Available from: https://www.gob.mx/salud/documentos/coronavirus-covid19-informe-tecnico-semanal

[5] Paediatric Intensive Care Society. PICS Statement: Increased number of reported cases of novel presentation of multisystem inflammatory disease. April 2020. Available from: https://pccsociety.uk/wp-content/uploads/2020/04/PICS-statement-re-novel-KD-C19-presentation-V2-27042020.pdf

[6] Morris SB, Schwartz NG, Patel P, Abbo L, Beauchamps L, Balan S, et al. Case series of multisystem inflammatory syndrome in adults associated with SARS-CoV-2 infection- United Kingdom and United States, March-August 2020. Morbidity and Mortality Weekly Report. 2020;**69**(40):1450-1456. DOI: 10.15585/mmwr.mm6940e1

[7] Centers for Disease Control and Prevention. Multisystem Inflammatory Syndrome in children (MIS-C) associated with Coronavirus Disease 2019 (COVID-19). 27 Mar 2020. Available from: https://emergency.cdc.gov/han/2020/han00432.asp

[8] World Health Organization. Multisystem Inflammatory Syndrome in children and adolescents temporally related to COVID-19. 2020. Available from: https://who.int/news-room/commentaries/detail/multisystem-inflammatory-syndrome-in-children-and-adolescents-with-covid-19

Section 1

Introduction

Chapter 1

Introductory Chapter: Multisystem Inflammation Syndrome

Nicolás Padilla-Raygoza and Gilberto Flores-Vargas

1. Introduction

Severe Acute Respiratory Syndrome Coronavirus (SARS-CoV-2), which caused Coronavirus Disease 2019 (COVID-19), emerged in late 2019 in Wuhan, China [1, 2], and has spread to virtually the entire world.

The infection has had a higher impact on older populations (over 40 years of age) and men. For example, Padilla et al. [3] reported that in Mexico, 58.48% of confirmed cases were men, and 97% were over 20 years old. Children and adolescents are susceptible to SARS-CoV-2 infection but usually develop COVID-19 at lower rates than adults, and the disease is less severe [4, 5].

In April 2020, the United Kingdom reported an increase in children with hyper-inflammatory shock and evidence of infection by SARS-CoV-2. This condition was named Multisystem Inflammatory Syndrome (MIS) [6]. MIS has been described in adults as a complication due to COVID-19 [7].

From there, cases of my children and adults have been reported in many countries [8, 9].

The incidence of MIS in children is estimated to be between 0.05% and 0.1% of those previously infected by SARS-CoV-2. A recent review study has revealed that most of the children with MIS (95.21%) recovered, while only 1–4% died from this syndrome [10, 11].

By January 2021, 6431 cases of MIS in children were reported. Of them, 55 died. 60% were Hispanic or Black [12].

Multiple organizations, including the CDC and the WHO, have proposed MIS case definitions. However, there is no test for the MIS diagnosis [7, 11, 13].

With the emergence of a hyperinflammation state in patients with COVID-19, Kawasaki's disease, severe macrophage activation syndrome, and systemic vasculitis with cardiomyopathy were considered for diagnosis [14–16]. Nevertheless, there are differences between MIS and those syndromes [17].

The emergence of SARS-COV-2 and COVID-19 has been a difficult situation for all countries. The emergence of new processes, such as MIS or the post-COVID-19 condition, is a current threat to health personnel and services.

2. Primary care. First level. Sanitary education and health promotion

Some recommendations against SARS-COV-2 infection were to use a facemask, to isolate COVID-19 cases for 10 days, to go out only for indispensable, hand washing, If you cough or sneeze cover mouth and nose with the elbow fold and social distancing

IntechOpen

(1 m or more) [18]. Nevertheless, many persons did not apply these measures, causing quick COVID-19 dissemination.

Besides, at a social level, schools were closed, and outdoor events were forbidden in most countries.

3. Second level. Specific protection

Due to the vaccination against SARS-COV-2, the frequency and severity of the disease decreased. Even so, there is much more to know about the current vaccines. It is worth noting that they were approved for emergency use.

4. Natural history of disease and prevention levels

The decision to address the natural history of the disease was motivated because it allowed us to review the disease's evolution and get some insight on how to prevent it. It also lets us compare MIS with previously detected and treated diseases.

The natural history model of the disease was developed in 1953 [19]. It establishes that disease results from a dynamic process that changes with time, space, and the person. There are factors that affect interactions between agents and guests. A preventive attitude should be developed [20].

The prepathogenic period, or ecological triad, is when the disease is absent, when the agent, the susceptible guest, and the environment are in equilibrium. If the balance is lost, the subclinical stage of the pathogenic period comes, where all the pathophysiological changes occurring in the body are described. In this period, the disease begins but does not yet manifest clinically. When signs and symptoms appear, the disease exceeds the clinical horizon. If the disease follows its natural course, complications will be presented or self-limited and return to the susceptible state, or can die. If the complications persist, the sequelae appear [20].

Regarding the levels of prevention, the prepathogenic period would correspond to the primary prevention, which has two levels. The first one is health education and health promotion, which would be all the activities to carry out so that the ecological

Prepathogenic period		**Pathogenic period**		
Agent Host Environment		Clinical	Complications	→ Recovery → Death → Sequelae
		Subclinical stage		
Primary prevention		Secondary prevention		Tertiary prevention
Sanitary education and health promotion	Specific protection	Early diagnosis and timely treatment	Limitation of damage	Rehabilitation

Source: Taken and modified from Ref. [20].

Table 1.
Natural history of disease and prevention level scheme.

triad does not break its balance and the disease does not occur. The second level of prevention would be specific protection, such as by applying vaccines to prevent the disease from being presented. In the pathogenic period, secondary prevention corresponds to its third level, an early diagnosis and timely treatment, for example, by applying all the measures to cure the disease in the initial phases. The fourth level would be the damage limitation or complications treatment. Tertiary prevention has the fifth level, the rehabilitation of sequelae (**Table 1**).

5. Conclusion

MIS has been reported in many countries among children and adults. It is crucial to be informed about the characteristics of this disease. The natural history of the disease and its levels of prevention is an agile way to review all aspects of MIS in children and adults. In this book, we also address other aspects of the disease to portray the big picture of the situation.

Author details

Nicolás Padilla-Raygoza* and Gilberto Flores-Vargas
Department of Research and Technological Development, Institute of Public Health from Guanajuato State, México

*Address all correspondence to: npadillar@guanajuato.gob.mx

References

[1] World Health Organization. Rolling updates on coronavirus disease (COVID-19). 2020. Available from: https://www.who.int/emergencies/diseases/novel-coronavirus-2019/events-as-they-happen [Accessed: March 23, 2020]

[2] Carlos WG, De la Cruz C, Cao B, Pasnick S, Jamil S. Novel Wuhan (2019-CoV) coronavirus. American Journal of Respiratory and Critical Care Medicine. 2020;**201**(4):7-8. DOI: 10.1164/rccm.2014P7

[3] Padilla-Raygoza N, Vega-Jiménez OU, García-Juárez A, Gallardo-Luna MJ, Navarro-Olivos E, León-Verdín MG, et al. Effect of Co-morbidities on mortality from COVID-19 in Mexico: An ecological study. Biomedical & Pharmacology Journal. 2021;**14**(1):7-13. DOI: 10.13005/bpj/2095

[4] Mehta NS, Mytton OT, Mullins EWS, Fowler TA, Falconer CL, Murphy OB, et al. SARS-CoV-2 (COVID-19): What do we know about children? A systematic review. Clinical Infectious Diseases. 2020;**71**(9):2469-2479. DOI: 10.1093/cid/ciaa556

[5] Parri N, Lenge M, Buonsenso D. Children with COVID-19 in pediatric emergency departments in Italy. The New England Journal of Medicine. 2020;**383**(2):187-190. DOI: 10.1056/NEJMc2007617

[6] Paediatric Intensive Care Society. PICS Statement: Increased number of reported cases of novel presentation of multisystem inflammatory disease 2020. 2020. Available from: https://pccsociety.uk/wp-content/uploads/2020/04/PICS-statement-re-novel-KD-C19-presentation-V2-27042020.pdf

[7] Morris SB, Schwartz NG, Patel P, Abbo L, Beauchamps L, Balan S, et al. Case series of multisystem inflammatory syndrome in adults associated with SARS-CoV-2 infection- United Kingdom and United States, march-august 2020. MMWR. Morbidity and Mortality Weekly Report. 2020;**69**(40):1450-1456. DOI: 10.15585/mmwr.mm6940e1

[8] Moraleda C, Serna-Pascual M, Soriano-Arandes A, Simo S, Epalza C, Santos M, et al. Multi-inflammatory syndrome in children related to SARS-CoV-2 in Spain. Clinical Infectious Diseases. 2020;**72**:e397-e401. DOI: 10.1093/cid/ciaa1042

[9] Dufort EM, Koumans EH, Chow EJ, Rosenthal EM, Muse A, Rowlands J, et al. Multisystem inflammatory syndrome in children in New York state. The New England Journal of Medicine. 2020;**383**(4):347-358. DOI: 10.1056/NEJMoa2021756

[10] Ruvinsky S, Voto C, Roel M, Fustiñana A, Veliz N, Brizuela M. Multisystem inflammatory syndrome temporally related to COVID-19 in children from Latin America and the Caribbean region: A systematic review with a meta-analysis of data from regional surveillance systems. Frontiers in Pediatrics. 2022;**10**:881765. DOI: 10.3389/fped.2022.881765

[11] Centers for Disease Control and Prevention. Multisystem inflammatory syndrome in children (MIS-C) associated with coronavirus disease 2019 (COVID-19). 2020. Available from: https://emergency.cdc.gov/han/2020/han00432.asp. [Accessed: March 27, 2020]

[12] CDC. COVID-19 information for pediatric healthcare providers. 2021.

Available from: https://www.cdc.gov/coronavirus/2019-cov/hcp/pediatric-hcp.html

[13] World Health Organization. Multisystem Inflammatory Syndrome in children and adolescents temporally related to COVID-19. 2020. Available from: https://who.int/news-room/commentaries/detail/multisystem-inflammatory-syndrome-in-children-and-adolescents-with-covid-19

[14] Bukulmez H. Current understanding of multisystem inflammatory syndrome (MIS-C) following COVID-19 and its distinction from Kawakasi disease. Current Rheumatology Reports. 2021;**23**:58. DOI: 10.1007/s11926-021-01028-4

[15] Loomba RS, Villareal EG, Flores S. COVISD-19 and hyperinflammatory syndrome in children: Kawasaki disease with macrophage activation syndrome in disguise? Cureus. 2020;**12**(8):e9515. DOI: 10.7759/creus.9515

[16] Gkoutzourelas A, Bogdanos DP, Sakkas LI. Kawasaki disease and COVID-19. Mediterranean Journal of Rheumatology. 2020;**31**(Suppl. 2):268-274. DOI: 10.31138/mjr.31.3.268

[17] Riphagen S, Gomez X, Gonzalez-Martínez C, Wilkinson N, Theocharis P. Hyperinflammatory shock in children during COVID-19 pandemic. Lancet. 2020;**395**(10237):1607-1608. DOI: 10.1016/S0140-6736(20)31094-1

[18] World Health Organization. WHO updates COVID-19 guidelines on masks, treatments and patient care. 2023. Available from: https://www.who.int/news/item/13-01-2023-who-updates-covid-19-guidelines-on-masks-treatments-and-patient-care

[19] Leavell HR, Clark EG. Preventive Medicine for the Doctor in his Community. 3rd ed. Vol. XVII. New York: McGraw-Hill; 1965. pp. 471-480

[20] de García Alba García JE, Salcedo Rocha AL. Historia natural y social de la enfermedad. En: Martínez y Martínez R, Rivera Montero R, eds. Salud y Enfermedad Del Niño y Del Adolescente. 8ª ed. Vol. 1. México: Manual Moderno. pp. 23-38

Section 2

Prepathogenic Period

Chapter 2

Pre-Pathogenic Period of Multisystemic Inflammatory Syndrome: Ecological Triad

Nicolás Padilla-Raygoza, Faina Linkov, Gilberto Flores-Vargas, María de Jesús Gallardo-Luna, Efraín Navarro-Olivos and Francisco Javier Magos-Vázquez

Abstract

In this chapter, we discuss Multisystemic Inflammatory Syndrome in children and adults. We begin by mentioning the antecedents and the origin of this disease. We frame this chapter in the ecological triad scheme and present the agent, host, and environment. It is necessary to theorize the new health threats in this scheme, based on a primary health-care approach, to understand how to prevent or inform accordingly. Due to its novelty, this syndrome originated from the SARS-CoV-2 infection still poses many questions. Future directions of this work include understanding the pathogenesis of MIS, including its mechanisms, risk factors, and diversity of outcomes.

Keywords: MIS-C, MIS-A, agent, host, environment

1. Introduction

Severe Acute Respiratory Syndrome Coronavirus (SARS-CoV-2), which causes Coronavirus disease 2019 (COVID-19), emerged in late 2019 in Wuhan, China [1, 2] and has spread to virtually the entire world.

The infection has had a higher impact on older populations (over 40 years of age) and men. For example, Padilla et al. [3] reported that in Mexico, 58.48% of confirmed cases were men, and 97% were aged over 20 years. Children and adolescents are susceptible to SARS-CoV-2 infection but usually develop COVID-19 at lower rates than adults, and the disease is less severe [4, 5].

A fraction of children affected by COVID-19 develop a life-threatening state of hyperinflammation 4 to 6 weeks after the onset of SARS-CoV-2 infection. This condition has been named Multisystem Inflammation Syndrome (MIS-C) [6]. A similar syndrome has been reported in adults (MIS-A), albeit as a rare complication of COVID-19 [7].

MIS-C was initially reported in the United Kingdom in April 2020, where an increase in critically ill children with hyperinflammatory shock and evidence of

SARS-CoV-2 infection was described [8]. There are also reports in Spain [9] and New York, USA [10]. The United States Centers for Disease Control and Prevention (CDC) and the World Health Organization (WHO) developed definitions for this entity [7, 11, 12].

The incidence of Multisystem Inflammatory Syndrome (MIS) in children is estimated to be between 0.05 and 0.1% of children who have been infected with COVID-19. Recent review study has revealed that the majority of MIS cases in children (95.21%) fully recovered while only 1–4% died from this syndrome [13, 14].

Case definitions for MIS have been developed by multiple organizations, including CDC and WHO; however, there is no single test that can demonstrate the diagnosis of MIS [7, 11, 12].

Systemic inflammation is the pathophysiological key to SARS-CoV-2 infection, with a host whose pro-inflammatory cytokines are responsible for the cytokine surge [15]. **Table 1** shows the CDC and WHO definitions for MIS-C and MIS-A.

MIS-C occurs in children under 21 years of age with a fever of 1 or more days, with laboratory evidence of inflammation, and in hospitalized patients, with two or more organs involved (cardiac, renal, respiratory, hematological, gastrointestinal, dermatological, and neurological), excluding other causes and RT-PCR/antigen/serology for positive SARS-CoV-2 and COVID-19 within the previous 4 weeks [11].

MIS-A presents in persons that are 21 years of age or older, with laboratory evidence of inflammation, hospitalized with one or more extrapulmonary organs involved, presenting with hypotension or shock, thrombosis, cardiac involvement, thromboembolism, acute liver injury, exclusion of severe respiratory disease or from other causes, and RT-PCR/antigen/serology positive for SARS-CoV-2 in the previous 12 weeks [7]. It is suspected as an abnormal immune system response to SARS-CoV-2 infection [16], causing systemic vasculitis and multiple organ damage [17].

At the beginning of the pandemic (April 2020), it was reported as a condition like Kawasaki disease [16, 17].

	CDC Children [11]	**CDC Adults [7]**	**WHO Children [12]**
Age (years)	< 21	≥ 21	0 a 19
Fever	>1 day	Without comment	>3 days
COVID-19	Yes	Yes (previous 12 weeks)	Yes
Severe disease	Yes	Yes	No
Involvement of extrapulmonary organs	≥ 2	≥ 1 (Extrapulmonary)	≥ 2
Absence of respiratory affection	No	Yes	No
Severe inflammatory evidence by laboratory *	Yes	Yes	Yes
Hospitalization	Yes	Yes	No

**Elevated C-reactive protein, procalcitonin, D-dimer, serum ferritin, erythrocyte sedimentation rate, fibrinogen, interleukin-6.*
Source: Taken and modified from Refs. [7, 11, 12].

Table 1.
Definitions of multisystem inflammation syndrome in children and adults according to CDC and WHO.

2. Other hyperinflammation syndromes

The first MIS-C and MIS-A cases were confused or considered as Severe Macrophage Activation Syndrome (SMAS), systemic vasculitis with cardiomyopathy, or a disease like Kawasaki disease with coronary artery aneurysm [18].

2.1 Macrophage activation syndrome (MAS)

The erythrocyte sedimentation rate is high in COVID-19 and low in MAS; furthermore, splenomegaly is almost pathognomonic in MAS, whereas it is not detected in MIS-C and the cytokine storm is different in MAS and post-COVID-19 [19].

2.2 Immune complex vasculitis

In MIS-C, there is ischemia due to the occlusion of blood vessels by immune complexes, such as spike proteins and anti-spike immunoglobulins; similar vasculitis is seen in adenosine deaminase 2 deficiency [18].

2.3 Kawasaki disease

Cases of severe hyperinflammation syndrome in COVID-19, resembling Kawasaki disease [20], have been reported in the United Kingdom [21], Italy [22], Spain [9], and the USA [16].

One difference between Kawasaki disease and MIS-C is the significant post-febrile thrombocytosis and coronary artery involvement compared to the myocardial involvement seen in MIS-C [20]. Another difference is that the CDC definition of MIS-C does not include skin rash [11].

Patients with MIS-C could have coronary artery aneurysm. Nevertheless, in most of them, it resolves during MIS-C follow-up; in Kawasaki disease, coronary artery aneurysms are more common and persist longer [23].

A crucial difference is that patients with COVID-19 have gastrointestinal clinical features, usually absent in Kawasaki disease [24].

MIS-C cases showed more pronounced laboratory abnormalities than those reported in Kawasaki disease; in both, the CRP was elevated, and the ferritin levels were elevated but lower in Kawasaki disease [16]; ethnicity was predominant in Afro-Americans in MIS-C, while in Kawasaki disease, it was in Asian descent. Other differences were that the COVID-19 patient developed lymphopenia, decreased platelets, and low albumin levels, while Kawasaki disease did not develop lymphopenia and showed less severe thrombocytopenia [18].

3. Multisystemic Inflammatory Syndrome epidemiology

The prevalence of MIS-C has been estimated at 2 per 100,000 children [10]. Waves of MIS-C cases follow 4–6 weeks after peaks of adult COVID cases [25, 26]. By early January in 2021, 6431 cases of MIS-C had been detected in the United States of America, with 55 deaths [27]. The prevalence of MIS-A is even less clear, and the CDC definitions are used to differentiate MIS-C and MIS-A. Basically, evidence of COVID-19 in the previous 2 weeks, age < 21 years, fever, and respiratory disease in children and absence of fever or respiratory disease in adults [7, 11].

4. Ecological triad

4.1 Agent

The SARS-CoV-2 coronavirus belongs to the order Nidovirales, family Coronaviridae, and genus Betacoronavirus. It can cause Coronavirus disease (COVID-19). The entire population is susceptible, and the forms of transmission include person-to-person contact, as droplets expelled by coughing or sneezing [28, 29].

Aerosol particles may be another form of transmission. There is no evidence of vertical mother-to-child transmission [30].

Coronaviruses are enveloped non-segmented positive-sense RNA [25], and SARS-CoV-2, which causes COVID-19, uses the same receptor, angiotensin-converting enzyme 2, as SARS-CoV, which is expressed in cells from respiratory tract epithelium; is the seventh member of the Coronavirus family to infect humans, and is more infectious than SARS-CoV or the Middle East Respiratory Syndrome Coronavirus (MERS-CoV), since SARS-CoV-2 grows better in the respiratory tract [31].

Since the emergence of the pandemic, the different variants of SARS-CoV-2 have been classified; in December 2020, the Alpha variant with lineage B.1.1.7 was reported [32]. The Beta variant was detected in October 2020 in South Africa, and there was no evidence of increased mortality with this variant [33]. The Gamma variant was detected in Japan in January 2021, and this variant is associated with increased transmissibility and mortality [33, 34] The Delta variant was identified in early 2021 in India and has increased risk of transmissibility and reinfection and became the predominant variant [33, 34]. The Omicron variant was identified in South Africa in November 2021, becoming the most transmissible and dominant worldwide [33].

4.2 Host

Most of the detected cases of MIS-C or MIS-A in the United States were Hispanic or Black (60%) [35]. Evidence suggests that anti-SARS-CoV-2 vaccination makes MIS-C less common among vaccines [36].

Affected children are reported to be between the ages of 2 and 16 years and were previously healthy children with no underlying health conditions [37].

MIS-C differs from MIS-A. In MIS-C, children were generally healthy prior to SARS-CoV-2 infection, and COVID-19 was mild or asymptomatic [10, 17], and reported fever of 1 or more days, with more of one affected body organ, including the respiratory, laboratory data showing inflammation (C-reactive protein, procalcitonin, D-dimer, serum ferritin, erythrocyte sedimentation rate, fibrinogen and interleukin-6) [11, 12] and predominantly in males (73%) [35].

In MIS-A, those affected had underlying health conditions and a history of respiratory disease [7, 38, 39], and generally did not have respiratory involvement, and fever may or may not be reported, and had tested positive for SARS-CoV-2 in the previous 12 weeks, detected by RT-PCR or virus antigen detection [7]. The most common ethnicities reported in MIS-A were Asian (25.4%), Caucasian (23.6%), and Hispanic (21.8%) [40].

The host responds by forming autoantibodies, antibody recognition of viral antigens in infected cells, and hyperinflammatory response due to viral superantigens. It is considered that gender, genetic predisposition, and ethnicity may play a crucial role in the occurrence of the disease syndrome [41].

4.3 Environment

The vast majority of the cases of MIS-C and MIS-A have been reported in hospitalized patients. Nevertheless, it appears that it is not the hospital environment that triggers the syndrome but that they were hospitalized due to the severity of the SARS-CoV-2 infection.

According to the CDC's definition of MIS-A, one of the criteria is that the patient was hospitalized due to the severity of COVID-19 [7].

5. Conclusion and future directions

The Multisystemic Inflammatory Syndrome originated from the SARS-CoV-2 infection and was first reported in children. Nevertheless, it also appeared to affect adults. Some differences are noted in the chapter. Even as the environment was the hospitals, it may only be the consequence of the COVID-19 severity. As evidence piles up, we will have a clearer picture of this disease and its ecological triad.

Future directions of MIS research include:

- Understanding the pathogenesis of MIS, including its mechanisms, risk factors, and diversity of outcomes. This includes:
    - Immune system characteristics in reaction to SARS-CoV-2
    - The impact of the virus on body's response to disease and individual variation of response
    - An autoimmune response to the virus.
- Developing better diagnostic tools for the early detection and management of the disease. Currently, there is no single test that can definitively diagnose MIS.
- Developing effective treatments. Supportive care utilized today, such as fluids, electrolytes, and anti-inflammatory drugs, may not work for everyone. Ideally, effective treatments will target the underlying mechanism of MIS onset and prevent serious complications.
- Identifying risk factors for MIS-C and for MIS-A. Developing a risk profile of the people most likely to be impacted by MIS.
- Studying the long-term effects of MIS including heart problems, kidney problems, and neurological complications.

Author details

Nicolás Padilla-Raygoza[1*], Faina Linkov[2], Gilberto Flores-Vargas[2], María de Jesús Gallardo-Luna[2], Efraín Navarro-Olivos[3] and Francisco Javier Magos-Vázquez[4]

1 Department of Research and Technological Development, Institute of Public Health from Guanajuato State, Mexico

2 Department of Health Administration and Public Health, John G. Rangos Sr. School of Health Sciences, Duquesne University, United States of America

3 Directorate of Teaching and Research, Institute of Public Health from Guanajuato State, Mexico

4 General Directorate of Health Services, Institute of Public Health from Guanajuato State, Mexico

*Address all correspondence to: npadillar@guanajuato.gob.mx

References

[1] World Health Organization. Rolling updates on coronavirus disease (COVID-19). Update 23 March 2020. 2020. Available from: https://www.who.int/emergencies/diseases/novel-coronavirus-2019/events-as-they-happen

[2] Carlos WG, De la Cruz C, Cao B, Pasnick S, Jamil S. Novel Wuhan (2019-CoV) coronavirus. American Journal of Respiratory and Critical Care Medicine. 2020;**201**(4):7-8. DOI: 10.1164/rccm.2014P7

[3] Padilla-Raygoza N, Vega-Jiménez OU, García-Juárez A, Gallardo-Luna MJ, Navarro-Olivos E, León-Verdín MG, et al. Effect of Co-morbidities on mortality from COVID-19 in Mexico: An ecological study. Biomedical & Pharmacology Journal. 2021;**14**(1):7-13. DOI: 10.13005/bpj/2095

[4] Mehta NS, Mytton OT, Mullins EWS, Fowler TA, Falconer CL, Murphy OB, et al. SARS-CoV-2 (COVID-19): What do we know about children? A systematic review. Clinical Infectious Diseases. 2020;**71**(9):2469-2479. DOI: 10.1093/cid/ciaa556

[5] Parri N, Lenge M, Buonsenso D. Children with COVID-19 in pediatric emergency departments in Italy. The New England Journal of Medicine. 2020;**383**(2):187-190. DOI: 10.1056/NEJMc2007617

[6] Godfred-Cato S, Bryan B, Leung J, Oster ME, Conklin L, Abrams J, et al. COVID-19-associated multisystem inflammatory síndrome in children – United States. MMWR. Morbidity and Mortality Weekly Report. 2020;**69**(32):1074-1080. DOI: 10.15585/mmwr.mm6932e2

[7] Morris SB, Schwartz NG, Patel P, Abbo L, Beauchamps L, Balan S, et al. Case series of multisystem inflammatory syndrome in adults associated with SARS-CoV-2 infection- United Kingdom and United States, march-august 2020. MMWR. Morbidity and Mortality Weekly Report. 2020;**69**(40):1450-1456. DOI: 10.15585/mmwr.mm6940e1

[8] Paediatric Intensive Care Society. PICS Statement: Increased number of reported cases of novel presentation of multisystem inflammatory disease. 2020. April 2020. Available from: https://pccsociety.uk/wp-content/uploads/2020/04/PICS-statement-re-novel-KD-C19-presentation-V2-27042020.pdf

[9] Moraleda C, Serna-Pascual M, Soriano-Arandes A, Simo S, Epalza C, Santos M, et al. Multi-inflammatory syndrome in children related to SARS-CoV-2 in Spain. Clinical Infectious Diseases. 2020;**72**:e397-e401. DOI: 10.1093/cid/ciaa1042

[10] Dufort EM, Koumans EH, Chow EJ, Rosenthal EM, Muse A, Rowlands J, et al. Multisystem inflammatory syndrome in children in New York state. The New England Journal of Medicine. 2020;**383**(4):347-358. DOI: 10.1056/NEJMoa2021756

[11] Centers for Disease Control and Prevention. Multisystem inflammatory syndrome in children (MIS-C) associated with coronavirus disease 2019 (COVID-19). 2020. Available from: https://emergency.cdc.gov/han/2020/han00432.asp

[12] World Health Organization. Multisystem Inflammatory Syndrome in children and adolescents temporally

related to COVID-19. 2020. Available from: https://who.int/news-room/commentaries/detail/multisystem-inflammatory-syndrome-in-children-and-adolescents-with-covid-19

[13] Ruvinsky S, Voto C, Roel M, Fustiñana A, Veliz N, Brizuela M. Multisystem inflammatory syndrome temporally related to COVID-19 in children from Latin America and the Caribbean region: A systematic review with a meta-analysis of data from regional surveillance systems. Frontiers in Pediatrics. 2022;**10**:881765. DOI: 10.3389/fped.2022.881765

[14] Patel JM. Multisystem inflammatory syndrome in children (MIS-C). Current Allergy and Asthma Reports. 2022;**22**:53-60. DOI: 10.1007/s11882-022-01031-4

[15] Ramos-Casals M, Brito-Zerón P, Marriette X. Systemic and organ-specific immune-related manifestations of COVID-19. Nature Reviews. Rheumatology. 2021;**17**:315-332. DOI: 10.1038/s41584-021-00608-z

[16] Cheung EW, Zachariah P, Gorelik M, Boneparth A, Kernie SG, Orange JS, et al. Multisystem inflammatory síndrome related to COVID-19 in previously healthy children and adolescents in New York city. Journal of the American Medical Association. 2020;**324**(3):294-296. DOI: 10.1001/jama.2020.10374

[17] Behzadi F, Ulloa NA, Danckers M. Multisystem inflammatory síndrome in adults: A case report and review of the literature. Journal of Medical Case Reports. 2022;**16**:102. DOI: 10.1186/s13256-022-03295-w

[18] Bukulmez H. Current understanding of multisystem inflammatory syndrome (MIS-C) following COVID-19 and its distinction from Kawakasi disease. Current Rheumatology Reports. 2021;**23**:58. DOI: 10.1007/s11926-021-01028-4

[19] Loomba RS, Villareal EG, Flores S. COVISD-19 and hyperinflammatory syndrome in children: Kawasaki disease with macrophage activation syndrome in disguise? Cureus. 2020;**12**(8):e9515. DOI: 10.7759/creus.9515

[20] Gkoutzourelas A, Bogdanos DP, Sakkas LI. Kawasaki disease and COVID-19. Mediterranean Journal of Rheumatology. 2020;**31**(Suppl. 2):268-274. DOI: 10.31138/mjr.31.3.268

[21] Riphagen S, Gomez X, Gonzalez-Martínez C, Wilkinson N, Theocharis P. Hyperinflammatory shock in children during COVID-19 pandemic. Lancet. 2020;**395**(10237):1607-1608. DOI: 10.1016/S0140-6736(20)31094-1

[22] Verdoni L, Mazza A, Gervasoni A, Martelli L, Ruggeri M, Ciuffreda M, et al. An outbreak of severe Kawasaki-like disease at the Italian epicentre of the SARS-CoV-2 epidemic: An observational cohort study. Lancet. 2020;**395**(10239):1771-1778. DOI: 10.1016/S0140-6736(20)31103-X

[23] Rowley AH, Shulman ST, Arditi M. Immune pathogenesis of COVID-19-related multisystem inflammatory syndrome in children. Journal of Clinical Investigation. 2020;**130**:5619-5621. DOI: 10.1172/JCI143840

[24] Bar-Meir M, Guri A, Godfrey ME, Shack AR, Hashkes PJ, Goldzweig O, et al. Characterizing the differences between multisystem inflammatory syndrome in children and Kawasaki disease. Scientific Reports. 2021;**11**:13840. DOI: 10.1038/s41598-021-93389-0

[25] Feldestein LR, Rose EB, Horwitz SM, Collins JP, Newhams MM, Son MBF, et al.

Multisystem inflammatory syndrome in U.S. children and adolescents. The New England Journal of Medicine. 2020;**383**(4):334-346. DOI: 10.1056/NEJMoa2021680

[26] Centers of Disease Control. COVID-19 information for pediatric healthcare providers. 2021. Available from: https://www.cdc.gov/coronavirus/2019-ncov/hcp/pediatric-hcp.html

[27] Li Q, Guan X, Wu P, Wang X, Zohu L, Tong Y, et al. Early transmission dynamics in Wuhan, China, of novel coronavirus infected pneumonia. The New England Journal of Medicine. 27 March 2020;**382**:1199-1207. DOI: 10.1056//NEJMoa2001316

[28] Munster VJ, Koopmans M, van Doremalen N, van Riel D, de Wit E. A novel coronavirus emerging in Chinakey questions for impact assessment. The New England Journal of Medicine. 2020;**382**(8):692-694. DOI: 10.1056/NEJMp2000929

[29] Zhu H, Wang L, Fang C, Peng S, Zhang L, Chang G, et al. Clinical analyses 10 neonates born to mothers with 2019-nCoV pneumonia. Translational Pediatrics. 2020;**9**:51-60. DOI: 10.21037/tp.2020.02.06

[30] Richman DD, Whitley RJ, Hayden FG, editors. Clinical Virology. 4a ed. Washington: ASM Press; 2016

[31] Zhu N, Zhang D, Wang W, Li X, Yang B, Song J, et al. A novel coronavirus from patients with pneumonia in China 2019. The New England Journal of Medicine. 2020;**382**(8):727-733. DOI: 10-1056/NEJMoa2001017

[32] Zárate S, Taboada B, Muñoz-Medina JE, Iša P, Sanchez-Flores A, Boukadida C, et al. The alpha variant (B.1.1.7) of SARS-CoV-2 failed to become dominant in Mexico. Microbiology Spectrum [Internet]. 2022;**10**(2):e0224021. DOI: 10.1128/spectrum.02240-21

[33] Chen KK, Tsung-Ning Huang D, Huang LM. SARS-CoV-2 variants - evolution, spike protein, and vaccines. Biomedical Journal. 2022;**45**(4):573-579. DOI: 10.1016/j.bj.2022.04.006

[34] Zhang Y, Zhang H, Zhang W. SARS-CoV-2 variants, immune escape, and countermeasures. Frontiers in Medicine. 2022;**16**(2):196-207. DOI: 10.1007/s11684-021-0906-x

[35] Centers of Disease Control. Multisystem inflammatory syndrome in children (MIS-C) in the United States. 2021. Available from: https://covid-cdc.gov/covid-data-tracker/#mis-national--surveillance

[36] Zambrana LD, Newhams MM, Olson SM, Halasa NB, Am P, Boom JA, et al. Effectiveness of Bnt162b2(Pfizer-Biontech)mRNA vaccination against multisystem inflammatory syndrome in children among persons aged 12-18 years-United States-July-December 2021. MMWR. Morbidity and Mortality Weekly Report. 2022;**71**:52-58. DOI: 10.15585/mmwr.mm7102e1

[37] Nakra NA, Blumberg DA, Herrera Guerra A, Lakshminrusimha S. Multisystem inflammatory syndrome in children (MIS-C) following SARS-CoV-2 infections: Review of clinical presentation, hypothetical pathogenesis, and proposed management. Children. 2020;**7**:69. DOI: 10.3390/children7070069

[38] Kunal S, Ish P, Sakthivel P, Malhotra N, Gupta K. The emerging threat of multisystem inflammatory syndrome in adults (MIS-A) in COVID-19: A systematic review. Heart &

Lung. 2022;**54**:7-18. DOI: 10.1016/j.hrtlng.2022.03.007

[39] Weatherhhead JE, Clark E, Vogel TP, Atmar RL, Kulkarni PA. Inflammatory syndromes associated with SARS-CoV-2 infection: Dysregulation of the immune response across the age spectrum. The Journal of Clinical Investigation. 2020;**130**(12):6194-6197. DOI: 10.1172/JCI145301

[40] Most ZM, Hendren N, Drazner MH, Perl TM. The striking similarities of multisystem inflammatory syndrome in children and a myocarditis-like syndrome in adults: Overlapping manifestations of COVID-19. Circulation. 2020;**143**(1):4-6. DOI: 10.1161/circulationaha.120.050166

[41] Marzano AV, Cassano N, Moltrasio C, Verdoni L, Genovese G, Vena GA. Multisystem inflammatory syndrome in children associated with COVID-19: A review with an emphasis on mucocutaneous and Kawasaki disease-like findings. Dermatology. 2021:1-9. DOI: 10.1159/000515449

Section 3

Clinical Stage

Chapter 3

Basic Mechanisms of Multisystemic Inflammatory Syndrome and Severe Acute Respiratory Syndrome Coronavirus 2

Cuauhtémoc Sandoval Salazar,
Paola Trinidad Villalobos Gútierrez,
Oscar Gútierrez Coronado and Vicente Beltrán Campos

Abstract

Multisystemic inflammatory syndrome is a condition developed by various factors such as chronic diseases, diverse body traumas, postoperative complications, and hypoxia. Within the main characteristics of this pathological condition, there is an increase in body temperature, free radicals, proinflammatory cytokines, lymphocytes, and even apoptosis. However, gravity depends on each of the organisms, its characteristics, as well as from the presence of other conditions such as overweight, obesity, and in recent years the infection has al severe acute respiratory syndrome coronavirus 2 (SARS-CoV-2), etc. With the above, it is essential to mention that the body uses several cell and molecular mechanisms to counteract the effects of inflammation for a long time. Therefore, life expectancy will depend on each patient's genetic, metabolic, and physiological response characteristics. This chapter describes the basic mechanisms given during the development of multisystemic inflammatory syndrome.

Keywords: inflammation, cytokines, SARS-CoV-2, immune system, multisystemic inflammatory syndrome

1. Introduction

Inflammation is a pathological process characterized by injury or tissue destruction caused by various cytologic and chemical reactions and usually manifested by typical signs of pain, heat, redness, swelling, and loss of function [1]. Aggressive factors such as a blow, exposure to toxic substances, lack of oxygen, and even autoimmune diseases generate inflammation. In general, during the inflammatory process, the organism develops a homeostatic regulation response to not alter or deregulate other essential basic functions of the cells, tissues, systems, or organs near the site of inflammation [2].

In cells and tissues, inflammation in principle facilitates the activation and participation of peptides and non-peptide molecules mediating the process, such as histamine, bradykinin, eicosanoids, chemokines, platelet-activating factor, fibrin, and the complement system. Subsequently, and once the process has begun, other cellular components of a protein nature will participate, such as proinflammatory cytokines or interleukins 1, 6 (IL-1, IL-6), tumor necrosis factor (TNF), as well as other attractant molecules such as interleukins 2, 8 (IL-8). The latter will induce the lymphocyte response; continuing with the inflammatory process, interleukin 3 (IL-3), granulocyte, and macrophage colony-stimulating factor (GM-CSF) will facilitate cell mitosis in the bone marrow. Finally, and in general, the inflammatory process is suppressed with interleukin 10 (IL-10) participation and transforming growth factor beta (TGF-β) [3].

In addition to the participation of the molecules mentioned above, other processes involve the increase of vascular diameter, thus facilitating blood flow to the affected area, followed by the elevation of temperature and redness. Subsequently, vascular permeability will increase, enabling the passage of fluid and immunoglobulin proteins that will generate edema. Finally, if the response to the acute inflammation is successful, the factor that caused the inflammatory process will be effectively eliminated and repaired; however, if the cell is functional or the damage is limited, the inflammation will continue and become a chronic or systemic event [4].

The main characteristic of systemic inflammation is the increase in the levels of inflammatory cytokines, as well as a more significant infiltration of macrophages to peripheral tissues. In this regard, this type of inflammation is considered a low grade, which is characteristic of maintaining the functionality of the affected tissue, for example, the inflammation present in diseases such as obesity, cardiometabolic, and other metabolic disorders, etc. [5].

On the other hand, there are also inflammatory processes such as Multisystemic Inflammatory Syndrome (MIS). The researchers detected this rare inflammation in children and adolescents infected with SARS-CoV-2; however, this condition has also developed in adults infected with SARS-CoV-2. The main characteristic of MIS is the development of inflammation in the whole organism. Therefore, the inflammatory process is in external and internal areas such as the heart, digestive system, skin, and brain. Moreover, this syndrome is more frequent in children than adults, who have been shown to recover faster from generalized inflammation and may not have severe cardiac complications [6].

2. Cellular mechanisms of inflammation

In the organism, the inflammatory process is complex because the factor that triggers it can be biological, chemical, or physical. As mentioned above, inflammation can be of acute and chronic type. The acute type has as its main characteristic the attraction of leukocytes due to the release of chemotactic molecules. The purpose of this action is to take care of the injury and specifically, the elimination of the agent that produced the activation of the inflammatory process and thus give way to regeneration or cellular repair [7].

During the acute phase, proinflammatory cytokines play a vital role. In this regard, all organism cells can synthesize and respond to these proteins, which vary in size (8–40,000 Da) and are soluble and pleiotropic. These molecules regulate other immune systems and blood-type cells' growth and functionality. In addition, given their distribution throughout the body, they have autocrine, paracrine and endocrine communication; and are classified according to the function they perform, but in general, their role is to mediate and regulate the processes of inflammation and immunity against aggressive stimuli that interrupt the inter and intracellular communication. It is essential to mention that there are several types of cytokines and among these are lymphokines, monokines and chemokines, which are produced by lymphocytes, monocytes and leukocytes [8].

In the acute phase of inflammation, platelets and granulocytic cells such as basophils, mast cells neutrophils and eosinophils; which are activated and, in turn, produce and release a series of soluble mediators that stimulate and regulate the inflammatory response. Initially, vasodilatation occurs due to increased blood flow to the affected area with the release of histamine and serotonin, followed by the participation of various molecules such as prostaglandins E (PGE1, PGE2), vasoactive intestinal polypeptide (VIP), bradykinin, and the complement system C5a and C3a. Then vascular permeability continues and in this process, in addition to the mediators PGE2, C5a and C3a, bradyB, kinin, leukotrienes B and D (LTB, LTD), fibrin products, neutrophil peptides, platelet-activating factor (PAF) and lymphokines are added. Subsequently, there is an infiltration of neutrophils by chemotaxis with the participation of C5a, LTB4, N-Formylmethionine (F-Met) peptides, PAF, IL-8, chemokines (CXCL1,2) and chemokine ligands (CCL3,4). After this comes the phase of macrophage involvement and the participation of other mediators such as lymphokines, glycopeptide (C5a desArg), fibronectin peptides, IFN, f-Met peptides, and monocyte chemoattractant protein (MCP-1). Finally, this process has two termination pathways; the first is to resolve the event of cell damage with the participation of inhibitory factors, enzyme inactivators (αM), free radical scavengers, TGF-β and IL-10. However, the other pathway allows the release of enzymes from the lysosome, an increase in free radicals and the participation of the IL-1 family group and TNFα, which will produce chronic or systemic inflammation [7].

Unlike acute inflammation, systemic inflammation is a progressive consequence that can culminate in multiple organ failure and death. During this process, inflammation is considered a non-specific defense mechanism with evident signs such as increases in body temperature, tachycardia, leukocytosis and tachypnea; for example, these manifestations are similar to those presented by patients with pancreatitis, severe trauma, severe burns, etc. In the physiopathology of systemic inflammation, the endothelium is the organ that maintains the inflammatory process; subsequently, systemic inflammation develops when various tissues are affected, either by injury, infection, hypoxia and increased free radicals or oxidative stress. In addition, as well as the participation of several molecules in the initial event of inflammation, in the systemic process participates, the nuclear factor Kappa-Beta (FN-kB), as well as its membrane receptors activated by active macrophage cytokines, virus free radicals, bacterial proteins, lipopolysaccharides and T lymphocytes [9]. Subsequently, once receptor activation has begun within the cytoplasm, protein kinases will phosphorylate and degrade the IFN-kB alpha inhibitor. With this, the heterodimer can target the cell nucleus and facilitate the translation of cytokines and other molecules involved in systemic inflammation. Another condition is the increase of free radicals, which will initiate a chain of intracellular events that will facilitate the release of the IFN-kB inhibitor; and then develop a positive regulation of genes that generate inflammatory proteins and increased production of molecules such as TNF, IL-2, serum activator proteins, nuclear factors, interleukins IL-1, IL-6, IL-8, nitric oxide synthase, lipid peroxidation, as well as a decrease in the endogenous antioxidant system and minerals such as selenium, zinc, and angiopoietins 1, 2 [9].

In addition to the above, the demanding need for protein synthesis produces deregulated metabolic modifications. For example, the nutrients in the body are distributed to all organs and systems to combat the inflammatory process. During this process, there is an increase in gluconeogenesis, proteolysis, lipolysis, lactic acid and oxide reduction processes to keep the immune system active and efficient. Unfortunately, during this process, the endogenous antioxidant capacity is overwhelmed, and generates oxidative stress; increases cellular damage, more cytokines are released, and reduces glutathione due to liver dysfunction. As described above, the maintenance of inflammation for too long develops systemic inflammatory syndrome and multiple organ failure (9).

2.1 The SARS-CoV-2 infection and the multisystemic inflammatory syndrome

During the Coronavirus disease (COVID-19) pandemic, there were initial complications in understanding the infection process and providing adequate pharmacologic treatment. Subsequently, with the application of vaccines, deaths and severe illnesses from the infection improved; however, in post-infection, children and adults developed an unexpected and not yet fully understood adverse condition, the multisystemic inflammatory syndrome MIS. This syndrome develops inflammation in various body parts, such as the gastrointestinal tract, heart and brain. This condition in children and adolescents infected by SARS-CoV-2 was detected initially; however, MIS can also develop in adults after infection and although it tends to be rare, it is severe [6]. The clinical manifestations of MIS in children are varied and have features representative of Kawasaki disease; for example, sepsis, toxic shock syndrome (TSS) and secondary hemophagocytic lymphohistiocytosis (sHLH). It is unknown to what extent children affected by MIS have a pathophysiology similar to this disease and to what time they might respond to the typical drugs used in these conditions and efficiently treated [10].

Continuing with what has been described above and specifically for SARS-CoV-2 infection, there is infection and replication of the virus in the cells and subsequently hyperinflammation develops. As is well known, the infection process requires the presence of receptors for angiotensin-converting enzyme 2; notably, the virus evades the immune response by suppressing IFN and interleukins IL-1, IL-6 and TNFα. This results in the multiplication of the virus inside the cell and its subsequent release when the cell dies and the viral load is released into the extracellular space, disperses and infects other cells. This condition will allow the activation of monocytes, neutrophils and the adaptive immune system mediated by T lymphocytes due to cellular damage and uncontrolled systemic inflammation [10]. In addition, a representative feature of SARS-CoV-2 infection is a cytokine storm or excessive and imbalanced stimulus release, in which there is excessive release of inflammatory molecules, leading to tissue and organ dysfunction and damage. Some of the signs and symptoms of this condition occur during the second-week post-SARS-CoV-2 infection, and signs and symptoms include fever, hypotension, rash, liver dysfunction, cytopenias, etc., as well as elevated IL-6 and IL-8 and other markers of inflammation. In this sense and as a differential factor from other viruses, SARS-CoV-2 infection has moderate ferritin increases, but the cytokine storm is more severe, associated with leukocytosis [11].

In addition to the above described, the increase of inflammation develops another phenomenon called antibody-dependent potentiation; this event facilitates the capture of viral detritus bound to immune cells in Fcc receptors, resulting in viral replication and organ damage. This phenomenon resembles dengue infection, where reinfections with a different serotype develop more severe clinical pictures. In the case of SARS-CoV-2 infected patients, there is a hypothesis that indicates that antibody-dependent potentiation may be critical in the development of severe infection, and the authors suggest that the process may be triggered by prior exposure to other SARS-CoV-2 serotypes, as well as common flew virus infections [12]. Notably, clinical manifestations in patients with this potentiation process include vasculitis (vasculitis skin lesions), microthrombi in small vessels and infarcts [13]. Finally and importantly, the maintenance process of the inflammatory state and presence of SARS-CoV-2 tends to be during 4 weeks and that antibody-dependent; these conditions indicate how the development of MIS starts from a delayed inflammation process [10].

Now, of the various molecules involved in the process of hyperinflammation, there are increases in ferritin, LDH, IL-6, IL-2, IL-10, TNF-α and decreases in lymphocytes (CD4, CD8), C-reactive protein, coagulation and abnormal renal function [14]. An important aspect to consider is that in the case of children, many presented mild symptoms of the infection and were even asymptomatic; this condition may predispose them to not providing specific and timely treatment, which could facilitate the worsening and severity of the disease [15]. Given the above, it is necessary to identify those signs and symptoms that indicate that people may have a severe MIS. To this end, specialists suggest the following aspects: first, there are the classic symptoms of the cardiac manifestations, such as dilated coronary arteries; then, as a second condition, there is sepsis, cardiovascular shock, or cardiac dysfunction. Similarly, the diagnosis considers a temperature higher than 38.5°C, skin rash, conjunctivitis, peripheral edema, severe abdominal pain, and diarrhea. In addition, although it may seem obvious, respiratory distress, in this case, is not one of the main symptoms. Other signs to identify are increased levels of procalcitonin, liver transaminases and anemia, thrombocytopenia or thrombocytosis, and the other molecules involved in hyperinflammation [16, 17]. Importantly, and potentially a confounding variable, not all patients are positive for SARS-CoV-2 by PCR but are positive for IgG antibodies. This feature indicates the likely hypothesis that MIS could represent a delayed inflammatory process [10].

2.2 Multisystemic inflammatory syndrome in children and adults

Given the complications that have occurred in the SARS-CoV-2 infected population during the COVID-19 pandemic, the development of MIS has been different according to age and has been more prevalent in children. In this regard, in 2021, a systematic review shows the signs and symptoms of multisystemic inflammatory syndrome in children. The main findings indicate that the median age of the affected children was 8 years, and among the signs and symptoms present during the infection were fever of more than 5 days in 99.4%, gastrointestinal problems (abdominal pain, vomiting, diarrhea) in 85.6%, cardiovascular problems (tachycardia, hemodynamic shock, myocarditis, coronary dilatation, etc.) in 79.3%, respiratory problems in 50.3% and increases in various inflammatory markers such as c-reactive protein, IL-6, and ferritin in 79.3%, respiratory problems in 50.3% and increases in inflammatory markers such as c-reactive protein, IL-6 and ferritin. Therefore, 73.3% of the patients were in intensive care but fortunately, only 1.9% of the total number of individuals presented mortality [18].

As previously described, after four to 6 weeks of SARS-CoV-2 infection and with a probable adaptive immune response, MIS develops; however, the pathophysiology is still unclear, given the diversity of signs and symptoms in patients. However, anti-SARS-CoV-2 antibodies, multisystem inflammation, cardiovascular and abdominal problems, and fever are widespread in children older than 5 years, although most pediatric patients are between 7 and 10 years of age. In this regard, many children present with MIS 36 to 45 days after initial symptoms due to COVID-19 [19]. In contrast to children infected with SARS-CoV-2 alone, children with SARS-CoV-2 who also developed MIS had increases in IL-17, IL-10 and TNF-α, and the authors indicate that this condition may be a post-infection sequela of COVID-19 and with a higher frequency of development in African Americans and Latinos [20].

Nevertheless, in the case of adults, the MIS is also complete since the signs and symptoms differ in each patient, so it is necessary to have a good knowledge of the condition and thus be able to give the appropriate treatment. As in infants, in the case of adults, symptoms include fever, rash, conjunctivitis, myocarditis and arrhythmias, fever, diarrhea, abdominal pain, myalgia, headache and some rare symptoms such as sore throat and chest pain; and in rare cases, vascular edema, ischemic/hemorrhagic stroke, status epilepticus, mononeuritis multiplex and thyroiditis; as well as, increases in c-reactive protein, IL-6 and positive serological values for SARS-CoV2 by serology or RT-PCR [21].

Therefore, the pathophysiology of MIS in adults is also still being determined. Several unproven hypotheses indicate that the main factors for its development include viral superantigens (e.g., 's-protein'), autoimmunity secondary to molecular mimicry with anti-Ro/La detectable in patients with MIS months after recovery, post-infection immune cell activation, and reservoirs of SARS-CoV2 infection still present [22]. However, the pathophysiology that favors the development of MIS is the activation and expansion of macrophages through antibody-dependent potentiation. Antibody-dependent potentiation is observed in multiple viral infections, including respiratory syncytial virus (RSV), measles and, most importantly, dengue virus, where it is thought to underpin the pathogenesis of dengue hemorrhagic fever. The antibody-dependent potentiation mechanism occurs following interaction with pre-existing non-neutralizing antibodies and virus binding and Fc Gamma receptor interaction during viral uptake in phagocytes, which facilitates viral proliferation and the release of proinflammatory cytokines, as well as the development of immune complexes that enhance the inflammatory process. While antibody-dependent potentiation has not been seen clinically in patients with SARS-CoV2 reinfection by different strains, it may occur due to the progressive changes observed within the S protein of different SARS-CoV-2 strains. It may also explain the link between vaccination and the development of MIS in adults [23].

Thus, although less common, adult MIS adds to a growing list of hyperinflammatory syndromes, each of which can be complicated and secondary to SARS-CoV2 infection, including secondary hemophagocytic lymphohistiocytosis and capillary leak syndrome [21]. For example in a hospital, a 22-year-old patient vaccinated against SARS-CoV-2 and 3 weeks after recovering from COVID-19 was admitted with a fever of 40.5oC, myalgias, headache and vomiting. The biochemical parameters showed neutrophilia (93.2%), thrombocytopenia (3.30%) and platelets in 51 × 109/L. Unfortunately, there was no accurate diagnosis with routine examinations, so the patient's condition worsened. Subsequently, the possible development of MIS was indicated and confirmed by increases in inflammation markers, Elevated CRP, Erythrocyte sedimentation rate, ferritin, procalcitonin, as well as elevated Troponin T, and myocarditis through ECG electrocardiogram and SARS-CoV-2 infection. With these data, the patient receives the appropriate treatment based on broad-spectrum antibiotics, corticosteroids, intravenous immunoglobulins, colchicine, and heparin [21].

3. Conclusions

The development of MIS has an interval of onset of 2–6 weeks and in some cases, there may be manifestation in the acute phase of SARS-CoV-2 infection; however, the latter is not evident since specialists agree that it may be due to the critical process or a post-infectious condition. It is essential to mention that MIS is a dangerous pathophysiological condition independent of whether the subject has has received the vaccine since factors such as genetic predisposition and comorbidities may be intrinsic in its development. Researchers agree that MIS is due to an active and prepared immune system through antibodies. The above, because the pharmacological treatment is directed at the immune system. Unfortunately, individual clinical studies are not sufficient to understand the pathophysiology of MIS, and at the same time, to provide effective treatment and follow-up to patients who have developed MIS. Another aspect to consider is the risk of relapse in MIS; therefore, randomized clinical studies are required to clarify the disease more efficiently. Finally, MIS is a complex condition that can develop after SARS-CoV-2 infection where the cellular physiology and clinical picture are still not understood.

Acknowledgements

We are grateful to the Universdad de Guanajuato, Campus Celaya-Salvatierra.

Conflict of interest

"The authors declare no conflict of interest."

Author details

Cuauhtémoc Sandoval Salazar[1*], Paola Trinidad Villalobos Gútierrez[2], Oscar Gútierrez Coronado[2] and Vicente Beltrán Campos[1]

1 División de Ciencias de la Salud e Ingenierias, Universidad de Guanajuato, Celaya, México

2 Centro Universitario de Los Lagos, Universidad de Guadalajara, Lagos de Moreno, Jalisco, Mexico

*Address all correspondence to: cuauhtemoc.sandoval@ugto.mx

References

[1] Medicine NLo. Inflammation. NIH-PUBMED2023. Available from: Inflammation - MeSH - NCBI (nih.gov). [Accessed: August 13, 2023]

[2] García BP. Inflamación. 2008 Revista de la Real Academia de Ciencias Exactas. Físicas y Naturales Serie A Matemáticas. 2008;**102**(1):91-159

[3] Suarez R, Buelvas N. Inflammasome: Activation mechanisms. Investigacion Clinica. 2015;**56**(1):74-99

[4] Vega Robledo GB. Inflamación. Revista de la Facultad de Medicina. National Autonomous University of Mexico. 2008;**51**(5):3

[5] Leon-Pedroza JI, Gonzalez-Tapia LA, del Olmo-Gil E, Castellanos-Rodriguez D, Escobedo G, Gonzalez-Chavez A. Low-grade systemic inflammation and the development of metabolic diseases: From the molecular evidence to the clinical practice. Cirugia Y Cirujanos. 2015;**83**(6):543-551

[6] CpecylPd E. Sindrome Inflamatorio Multisistémico. United State of America: CDC; 2023. Available from: Síndrome inflamatorio multisistémico en adultos (MIS-A, por sus siglas en inglés) (cdc.gov). [Accessed: August 13, 2023]

[7] Germolec DR, Shipkowski KA, POR F, Evans E. Markers of inflammation. In: DJ C, RC E, BC C, editors. Inmunotoxicity Testing Methods and Protocols. Second ed. Methods in Molecular Biology New York, NY: Humana Press; 2018. p. 22

[8] Khawar B, Abbasi MH, Sheikh N. A panoramic spectrum of complex interplay between the immune system and IL-32 during pathogenesis of various systemic infections and inflammation. European Journal of Medical Research. 2015;**20**:8

[9] Jesús DM. Síndrome de respuesta inflamatoria sistémica. Aspectos fisiopatológicos. Revista de la Asociación Mexicana de Medicina Crítica y Terapia Intensiva. 2009;**23**(4):9

[10] Tanner T, Wahezi DM. Hyperinflammation and the utility of immunomodulatory medications in children with COVID-19. Paediatric Respiratory Reviews. 2020;**35**:81-87

[11] Leverenz DL, Tarrant TK. Is the HScore useful in COVID-19? Lancet. 2020;**395**(10236):E83

[12] Francesco N. Is antibody-dependent enhancement playing a role in COVID-19 pathogenesis? Swiss Medical Weekly. 2020;**150**:4

[13] Felsenstein S, Herbert JA, McNamara PS, Hedrich CM. COVID-19: Immunology and treatment options. Clinical Immunology. 2020;**215**:13

[14] Moutchia J, Pokharel P, Kerri A, McGaw K, Uchai S, Nji M, et al. Clinical laboratory parameters associated with severe or critical novel coronavirus disease 2019 (COVID-19): A systematic review and meta-analysis. PLoS One. 2020;**15**(10):25

[15] Dong YY, Mo X, Hu YB, Qi X, Jiang F, Jiang ZY, et al. Epidemiology of COVID-19 among children in China. Pediatrics. 2020;**145**(6):10

[16] Riphagen S, Gomez X, Gonzalez-Martinez C, Wilkinson N, Theocharis P. Hyperinflammatory shock in children during COVID-19 pandemic. Lancet. 2020;**395**(10237):1607-1608

[17] Verdoni L, Mazza A, Gervasoni A, Martelli L, Ruggeri M, Ciuffreda M, et al. An outbreak of severe Kawasaki-like disease at the Italian epicentre of the SARS-CoV-2 epidemic: An observational cohort study. Lancet. 2020;**395**(10239):1771-1778

[18] Hoste L, Van Paemel R, Haerynck F. Multisystem inflammatory syndrome in children related to COVID-19: A systematic review. European Journal of Pediatrics. 2021;**180**(7):2019-2034

[19] Kabeerdoss J, Pilania RK, Karkhele R, Kumar TS, Danda D, Singh S. Severe COVID-19, multisystem inflammatory syndrome in children, and Kawasaki disease: Immunological mechanisms, clinical manifestations and management. Rheumatology International. 2021;**41**(1):19-32

[20] Diorio C, Henrickson SE, Vella LA, McNerney KO, Chase J, Burudpakdee C, et al. Multisystem inflammatory syndrome in children and COVID-19 are distinct presentations of SARS CoV-2. Journal of Clinical Investigation. 2020;**130**(11):5967-5975

[21] Worku D. Multisystem inflammatory syndrome in adults (MIS-A) and SARS-CoV2: An evolving relationship. BioMed. 2023;**2023**(3):6

[22] Lai C-C, Hsu C-K, Hsueh S-C, Yen M-Y, Ko W-C, Hsueh P-R. Multisystem inflammatory syndrome in adults: Characteristics, treatment, and outcomes. Journal of Medical Virology. 2023;**95**(2):e28426

[23] Shun IT, Tadaki A, Suzuki. Insights into pathology and pathogenesis of coronavirus disease 2019 from a histopathological and immunological perspective. JMA Journal. 2021;**4**(3):8

Chapter 4

Systemic Immune-Inflammatory Index and Other Inflammatory Markers in Odontogenic Cervicofacial Phlegmons

Ciprian Ioan Roi, Alexandra Roi and Mircea Riviș

Abstract

Odontogenic cervicofacial phlegmons represent a medical and surgical emergency, being characterized by a high mortality rate. The evolution of the infection toward the superficial and deep cervicofacial spaces is strongly related to the immune status of the individual. These complications are a challenge for the clinician, and a complete assessment of the case is mandatory. By integrating the value of the systemic immune-inflammatory index and other inflammatory markers determined from blood samples, a complete evaluation of the case can be provided from the beginning by assessing the individualized response of the immune system. The systemic immune-inflammatory index has proved its efficiency in assessing the relationship between the host's inflammatory and immunological condition by integrating the values of the neutrophils, platelets and lymphocytes. Also, the neutrophils-lymphocytes ratio (NLR) can be an important inflammatory marker for revealing the general expansion of the infection. The ongoing treatment and the response are important steps for the outcome of the cases. The quantification of the immune response through these parameters can efficiently guide the initial diagnosis, the treatment options, the continuous monitorization, and, eventually, the prognosis of the patients.

Keywords: odontogenic infections, cervicofacial phlegmons, inflammatory markers, systemic immune-inflammatory index, prognostic

1. Introduction

The odontogenic cervicofacial phlegmons represent an infection with an aggressive evolution toward the nearby anatomical spaces, both superficial and deep ones. Having as a main cause the odontogenic pathogens, their first localization could be in the tooth structures or the periodontium, having the ability to disseminate into the alveolar bone and surrounding soft tissue. Several conditions can influence the progression of oral pathogens, conditions that are represented by the incidence of complications after teeth exodontia, salivary glands pathologies, malignancies that involve the oral hard and soft tissue, and associated health problems of the patient. A concern related to this type of infection is its potential to progress along the facial planes, until, in severe cases, it affects the mediastinum, a situation that requires emergency management of the case, being a life-threatening complication. There are certain complications that the clinician must identify in order to assess the case correctly, and these complications can include internal jugular vein thrombosis, mediastinitis, arterial erosion, pneumonia, empyema, meningitis and sepsis. Special attention must be given to immunocompromised patients, as their immune system cannot manage properly the response to infection, and the delay of the treatment can influence the severity of the case. Normally, the oral cavity is populated with a specific oral flora, known as the oral microbiome, and in a healthy environment, all the pathogens are in symbiosis. Any perturbance in the balance of the oral microflora will determine the increase of specific microorganisms that will influence the occurrence of different pathologies [1–3].

The evolution of the cervical facial phlegmons is strongly influenced by the response of the immune system, outlining the importance of a prompt evaluation of the case and the existent correlation with existent comorbidities. Among the first evaluations of the patients, the assessment of the inflammatory response is mandatory, being a relevant prognostic value for the case. A helpful approach for these cases would be the permanent monitorization of several inflammation biomarkers identified in the blood, which could offer important information regarding the initial status of the patient, the response of the immune system in relationship with the polymicrobial infection and the evolution of the values of these biomarkers along with the initiation of the surgical treatment and medication.

A complete evaluation of the systemic immune-inflammatory index and other inflammatory markers in correlation with this type of severe infection could be an important step for the initial evaluation of the case, the management and response of the immune system along with the decided treatment option, and for the final evaluation that certifies the absence of the infection present in cervicofacial phlegmons.

Taking into consideration the severe evolution, bad prognosis and high mortality rate associated with these types of infections, the evaluation of the response of the immune system could be the key. Integrating a personalized analysis of these predictive systemic inflammation markers, the management of the clinical cases of odontogenic cervicofacial phlegmons and the survival rate could be improved.

This chapter aims to provide an overview of the odontogenic cervicofacial phlegmons, its causes and aggressive evolution, highlighting the potential that systemic immune-inflammatory index and several inflammatory biomarkers have in the management of the cases.

2. Cervicofacial phlegmons-etiology

2.1 Odontogenic causes

The periodontium, the alveolar bone, and the periosteum are the first oral structures affected by the pathogens and their toxins. Dental pulp gangrene and periodontal diseases are the main bacterial reservoirs capable of initiating odontogenic phlegmons. The route of bacteria dissemination is represented by the tooth crown destruction, dental pulp and tooth apex. After this pattern is followed, the pathogens can migrate into the soft tissues of the head and neck. The shape and anatomical characteristics of the neck and the head region affect the path that the inflammatory processes spread. Through continuity, the presence of blood and lymphatic vessels, as well as through the neurolemma, the infection advances from the oral cavity, face, and neck to the nearby anatomical areas represented by the superficial and deep fascial spaces [1]. The most involved teeth are the inferior molars, but the implication of the frontal teeth is not excluded [2, 3].

2.2 Microbial pathogens

The cervicofacial phlegmons are polymicrobial infections including intraoral indigenous bacteria. Viridans group streptococci and Staphylococcus aureus are the pathogens that are most commonly identified in patients with Ludwig angina, but anaerobes including Bacteroides, Prevotella, Fusobacterium, Peptostreptococci, and peptococci are also frequently implicated. The frequency of anaerobic infection increases with infection severity and dissemination [4, 5]. The infection with *Streptococcus anginosus,* which is a virulent strain from viridans group streptococci, or infection with gram-negative aerobic infection as well as methicillin-resistant *Staphylococcus aureus* (MRSA) is correlated with a bad prognosis [3]. In cases of patients with cervicofacial phlegmons and diabetes, the infection with Klebsiella was diagnosed in over half of the patients [6]. Routine aerobic and anaerobic cultures must be performed on samples of drained secretions of the phlegmons from the first presentation of the patient and successive in the case of unfavorable evolution of the cases. The result of the cultures must be correlated with the pharmacological antibiotherapy.

2.3 Nonodontogenic factors

The other factors that can be involved in the etiopathogeneses of the cervicofacial phlegmons are divided into:

- **local factors:** mandibular fractures, osteomyelitis, soft tissue laceration, sialadenitis, sialolithiasis of the submandibular glands, tumor superinfection, postoperative status, pharyngeal infections and tonsillitis, neoplasms, lingual piercing, foreign bodies, otitis media, peritonsillar abscess, iatrogenic, infectious lesions of the subcutaneous tissue (Staphylococcic infections, suppurated atheroma), superinfected cystic pathology of the thyroglossal tract, general dissemination of the infection, mastoiditis, traumatic penetration of oropharynx, lymphocele [7].

- **general factors:** systemic illnesses such as diabetes mellitus, mental illness, malnutrition, liver diseases, alcoholism, drug abuse, neutropenia, glomerulonephritis, and a compromised immune system (caused by AIDS, systemic lupus erythematosus, immunosuppression) [3, 8].

2.4 Dissemination routes

Regarding the anatomy of the mandibular alveolar bone, the submandibular space and the roots of the inferior molars that are adjacent, allowing dental infections that develop in the alveolar bone to spread in the submandibular space. The roots are situated below the mylohyoid muscle's insertion. In fact, this route of transition is the main explanation for the majority of phlegmons.

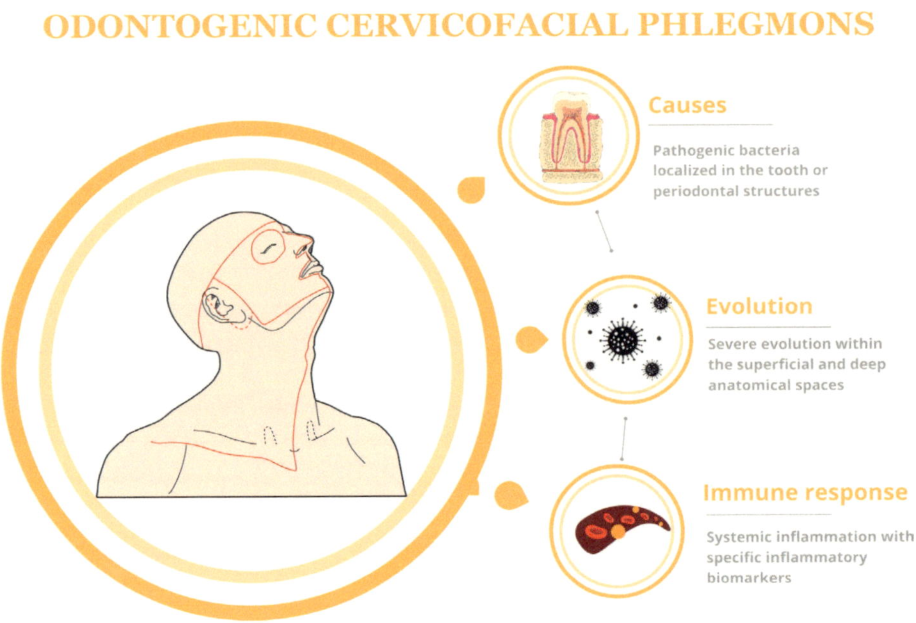

Figure 1.
Odontogenic cervicofacial phlegmons characteristics (personal design and propriety of the authors).

The spreading of the infection is favored by the natural connection between deep neck spaces. So, the infection can spread directly or in the lymphatic way. Additionally, inflammation spreads in the sublingual region, between the hyoglossus and genioglossus muscles, and involves the mylohyoid muscles area. The inflammation process gains access to the epiglottis in this manner, where it causes edema. The hyoid bone and the mandibular body prevent edema from spreading in other anatomic spaces. The edema and the cellulitis can be transmitted to the deep cervical fascia. The submandibular infection may descend to the mediastinum through the deep cervical fascia. The infection can, albeit less frequently, extend to the carotid, pterygopalatine region or cavernous sinus (**Figure 1**) [1, 3].

3. Clinical aspects

The classic inflammatory signs are present in the cervicofacial region: *rubor, tumor, dolor, calor, function laesa.* The first symptoms develop at a high speed and are represented by dental pain, hypersalivation, throat pain and otalgia in the early stages, followed by dysphagia, odynophagia, dysphonia, salivary gland secretion disorders and trismus [9–11].

3.1 Local examination

The teguments become livid and tense, glossy, few hyperemic areas, with increased consistency and are usually described as “woody”. The area of the neck is firm, edematous, very painful, described as nonfluctuating and without signs of pastiness. Cervical area of the neck is swollen, taking the aspect of” bull neck” and by deformity, the jawline is lost. Double chin aspect is also present as a consequence of the accumulation of the inflammatory exudate in that area. The saliva is drooling, and the patient has difficulty in speaking [12]. Open mouth, mandibular protrusion, and tongue lifted are all symptoms of these patients. Cervicofacial soft tissues may develop subcutaneous emphysema.

The edema is located bilateral and placed above the suprahyoid muscles. The muscle tonus is increased, the area has a nonfluctuating consistency, and the palpation in the affected region is painful. Usually, the patient's mouth is half open, and the tongue is in an elevated position, in contact with the hard palate, as a consequence of the oral floor edema. The described position of the tongue as superior and posterior can eventually lead to asphyxiation [12, 13].

3.2 General implications

General health status of the patients affected by cervicofacial phlegmons is influenced. In the first stages, the patient can present fever, chills, and general weakness. In a few hours, the symptoms advance in intensity and gravity, with the presence of meningismus, drooling, tachycardia, general agitation, respiratory distress, difficulty breathing, stridor, cyanosis of the teguments and mental alteration status [14]. Patients diagnosed with phlegmon of the oral floor often suffer from dehydration, partially caused by the limitations and pain during dysphagia or as a consequence of the high levels of toxicity in the bloodstream, fact that determines increased sweating and urination, leading to an abnormal general fluid loss [13].

Since hypoxia brought on by obstruction of superior airways is the primary cause of mortality in the first stages of cervicofacial phlegmons, maintaining the permeability of the patient's airways must be given top attention. The elevation of the oral floor and the posterior positioning of the tongue is a risk of obstruction of the airways. The edema of the epiglottis can also be present and can be a factor that explains the obstruction of the upper airways by blockage.

The edema and the phlegmon pathogens can progress, affecting the parapharyngeal space, and evolving toward the mediastinum, causing severe infections such as mediastinitis, pericarditis, bronchial erosions, and severe heart and pulmonary complications. Strenuous monitoring of the patients is required for any indications of airway blockages, such as stridor and the usage of supplementary breathing muscles. As symptoms worsen, patients may lean forward in the tripoding position in order to maximize the airway diameter. Oxygenation less than 94% associated with clinical signs of airway obstruction are indications for endotracheal intubation, tracheostomy or cricothyroidotomy. The severity of the symptoms requires rapid treatment and admission on ICU [15].

3.3 Complications

General complications can occur at multiple organs, are life-threatening and cand lead to exitus of patients with cervicofacial phlegmons:

- **cardiovascular system:** endocarditis, pericarditis, abscess of the carotid sheath and jugular thrombophlebitis, hematogenous dissemination to distant organs, coagulation abnormalities ranging from thrombocytopenia to a fulminant state of disseminated intravascular coagulation (DIC)

- **respiratory system:** pleuropulmonary suppuration, aspiration pneumonia, pneumothorax, descending mediastinitis
- **maxillofacial region**: necrotizing fasciitis, brain abscess, mandibular or cervical osteomyelitis, cavernous sinus thrombosis, Lemierre's Syndrome, orbital abcess.

4. Systemic inflammatory response

4.1 Generalities

A systemic inflammatory response from the host is triggered in response to a severe microbial infection of the cervicofacial spaces, as described in the cervicofacial phlegmons. This reaction appears as a response to limit the infection and minimize the general complications. The basic symptoms of this self-defense response that can be observed include fever, tachycardia, tachypnea, and hypotension.

The bacterial activity in the cervicofacial phlegmons leads to significant necrosis of the muscles. Anaerobic organisms are found isolated when the gangrene affects the surrounding soft tissues, as a consequence of the combined action of the hypoxia, released bacterial toxins and the effect of the interstitial pressure. The anaerobic organisms develop even in the soft tissues without gangrene. The tissue is described as being diffuse infiltrated with the presence of neutrophils and dead histiocytes. The presence of leukocytosis is usually described by the involvement of nuclear polymorphic leukocytes [16].

Inflammatory markers evaluated by blood tests are commonly used as objective evaluation parameters both at the admission of the patient, before the surgical and pharmacological treatment and after, in order to assess the gravity of the case and the efficiency of the treatment.

4.2 Immune system cells activity

The immune system, which is a combination of specialized cells that serves as a protective barrier and is made up of an innate system and an acquired system, mediates immunological response. When exposed to an antigen, the innate system launches a general defensive response. On the other hand, the acquired system is an antigen-specific defensive mechanism that has the ability to identify the antigen. As a result, memory cells are developed, and cand recognize and react to an antigen in the event of a new exposure [17].

Leukocytes, which include T, B, and killer lymphocytes, granulocytes, which include neutrophils, basophils, eosinophils, and mast cells; and antigen-presenting cells, which include macrophages, Langerhans cells, and dendritic cells, form the immune system. An immune response to infection is triggered by bacterial invasion. The macrophage is the organism's initial defense cell. It performs a dual role as an antigen-presenting cell to the neutrophils, who are in charge of bacterial phagocytosis, and as a releaser of chemotactic chemicals that draw them to the site of the lesion. Histamines, bradykinins, cytokines, and prostaglandins are released, which causes vasodilation and the opening of gaps between endothelial cells, enabling plasma to extravagate into the interstitial spaces where it collects and fibrin to develop [18].

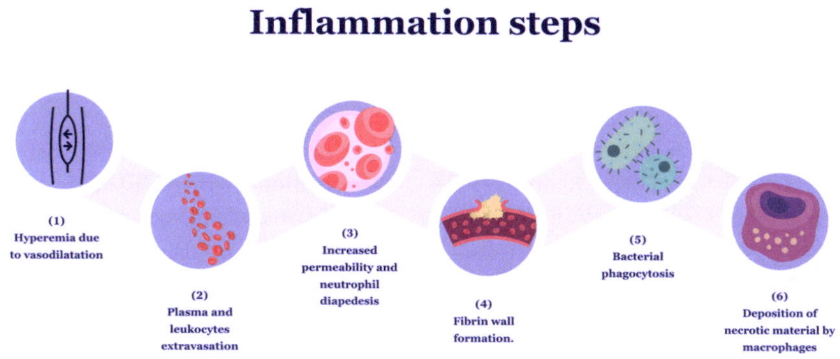

Figure 2.
Steps of the inflammation (personal design and propriety of the authors).

Bacterial invasion initiates a series of immunological reactions in order to eradicate the cervicofacial infection. The first fight is a defense process initiated by the macrophage cells. The macrophage has a dual role:

1. releasing chemotactic factors that attract neutrophils to the infection site

2. are an antigen-presenting cell to the neutrophils in order to perform bacterial phagocytosis.

The chemical mediators such as histamines, bradykinins, cytokines and prostaglandins are released. This process causes vasodilatation and widening of spaces between endothelial cells, allowing the plasma extravasation into the interstitial spaces where it accumulates, followed by the development and accumulation of fibrin (**Figure 2**) [19].

4.3 Systemic inflammatory response syndrome (SIRS)

SIRS is a progressive, pathophysiological process, being the first phase of the systemic host response to odontogenic infections. In the past, the combination of infection and SIRS was defined as sepsis. However, further studies showed that sepsis is not only a pro-inflammatory condition; it may also trigger an early anti-inflammatory reaction in the organism [20].

The reaction of the immune system can be described by two or more of the following conditions:

1. The body temperature under 36.0°C and/or over 38.0°C

2. The heart rate is modified, over 90 beats/minute

3. The respiratory rate is increased, being over 20 breaths/minute or the PaCO2 under 32 mmHg

4. The white blood cell count is over 12,000/cumm, under 4000/cumm, or over 10% immature (band) forms present [21]

5. Inflammatory biomarkers

5.1 Generalities

The commonly used markers for assessing the inflammatory activity of the organisms are the C-reactive protein (CRP), the procalcitonin (PCT), the modified white blood cell count (WBC) and its fractions (neutrophils, lymphocytes and monocytes). However, their values individually cannot determine exactly the severity of the cervicofacial phlegmon cases [22].

5.2 C-reactive protein (CRP)

The C-reactive protein is frequently used as a marker of the presence of inflammation in the organism. Its values are taken into consideration during the diagnosis of head and neck infection detection. However, because it speaks about two days after infection begins, it may not always reflect real-time illness disease [23, 24]. When infection is suspected, CRP is typically evaluated at the time of admission of the patient to the hospital. It can be measured objectively and consistently throughout time. Daily monitoring is more sensitive than body temperature or white blood cell count in the identification of sepsis [25].

Less than 1 mg/L of CRP is considered to be normal. After being stimulated by interleukin-6 (IL-6), its level rises within the first 6 hours and can reach a peak level of around 350–400 mg/L after about 48 hours. Its half-life is between 20 and 24 hours [26].

It is generally accepted that CRP rise in the 10–40 mg/L range is brought on by viral infections and moderate inflammation. CRP levels range from 40 to 200 mg/L when there is active inflammation and bacterial infection. Burns and severe bacterial infections as cervicofacial phlegmons have levels above 200 mg/L.

5.3 Procalcitonin (PCT)

PCT, a precursor of calcitonin, is produced by the thyroid gland's C-cells. Additionally, PCT is secreted as a result of an immune system response to endotoxins and a mediated response to bacterial infections. For predicting systemic bacterial inflammation, PCT has the best sensitivity and specificity. PCT is considered to have a higher diagnostic value compared to the other traditional tests, among which are the C-reactive protein levels, the white blood cell count, and the levels of interleukin (IL)-6. PCT levels can be used to decide when to start and how long to take antibiotic therapy since they are related to how serious bacterial infections are. In order to swiftly assess a patient's systemic infection status and begin therapy, PCT analysis may be completed quickly [27].

Serum PCT concentration in healthy individuals is typically <0.1 ng/mL. The absence of bacterial infection is not necessarily indicated by a low or normal PCT content.

This could be the case, notably, during the first stages of bacterial infections or in localized infections. When bacterial infection is present, PCT rises, and the magnitude of the high levels is inversely correlated with the severity of the illness. Patients are more likely to develop a systemic infection if their PCT levels are higher than 0.5 ng/mL. Comparatively to patients with broad sepsis, severe sepsis, and septic shock like patients diagnosed with cervicofacial phlegmons, patients with localized infections have lesser increases in PCT. PCT was confirmed to be a highly accurate test for diagnosing sepsis in patients with maxillofacial infections [20, 27, 28].

5.4 Prepesin (PSEP)

Prepesin represents a specific high-affinity receptor for the lipopolysaccharide (LPS), CD14 being a cell surface antigen cluster marker protein found on neutrophils and monocytes. It is produced by the bone marrow cells and is described as a fragment of CD14. It engages with LPS and then proceeds through a number of signaling pathways and immunological chain reactions. CD14 can be encountered as bound to a membrane CD14 and as a soluble CD14 (sCD14). In case of several pathologies, such as the presence of sepsis, the syndrome of acute respiratory distress, lupus erythematous and the acquired immunodeficiency syndrome, elevated plasmatic concentrations have been reported in case of sCD14 [29].

Although sCD14 functions as a common coreceptor, it is not a specific marker of sepsis on odontogenic infections. Because of this, only the sCD14 subtype, that represents a fragment of CD14 that is released from the bloodstream, with the property of binding to a bacterial pathogen that is related to a specific bacterial infection. It was initially identified during the CD14 reaction, and studies afterward characterized it as a specific marker for the presence of bacterial infections. The epidemiological and molecular aspects of PSEP are still not well understood. The sCD14 subtype levels in the plasma samples were determined using an enzyme immunoassay (EIA), and is known as prepesin [29].

Patients diagnosed with severe cervicofacial phlegmons, the plasma levels of PSEP increase faster than C-reactive protein or procalcitonin levels, the PSEP increased levels can be detected within 4 h of infection. Moreover, the determination time is significantly short (20 min) compared to the other inflammation biomarkers. PSEP can be successfully used for the diagnosis and quantification of the severity of the odontogenic infections and systemic status of the patients. Also, it can be combined with other existing diagnostic approaches for a proper evaluation of the case prognosis.

5.5 White blood cells (WBC)

The white blood cell count (WBC) and its representative fractions (neutrophils, monocytes and lymphocytes) are often used at hospital admission of the patients with cervicofacial phlegmons. However, their determined values alone cannot represent an indicator for the severity of the infection or the prognosis of the odontogenic suppuration cases [30].

6. New prognosis inflammatory indicators

6.1 Systemic immune-inflammation index (SII)

It is a new paraclinical analysis that assesses systemic inflammation and uses the patient's inflammatory biomarkers. This index is calculated based on the following formula: (N × P)/L (N, P, and L represent neutrophils, platelets, and lymphocytes, respectively)-**Figure 3**. The SII is a novel inflammatory biomarker that can evaluate the prognosis in a wide range of diseases, including solid malignant tumors, pulmonary

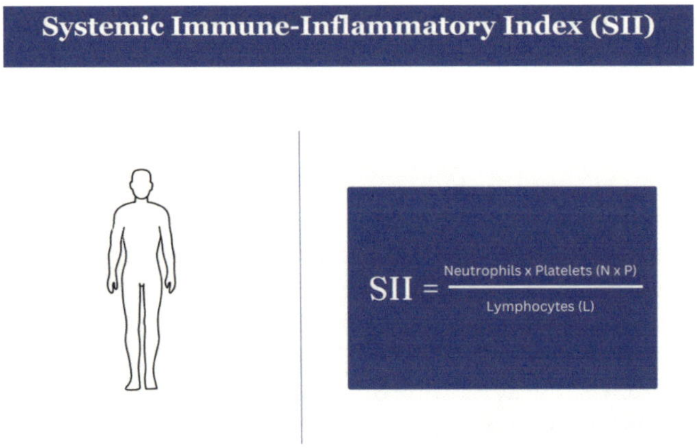

Figure 3.
SII formula (personal design and propriety of the authors).

embolism, and coronary artery diseases [31]. For SII determination, antecubital venous blood must be collected, and a routine blood examination must be performed immediately after the blood sample is collected. It is a rapid and precise determination, and the results can guide the practician regarding the inflammatory status of the cases.

The distinctions between the functions of lymphocytes, neutrophils, and platelets throughout the immune response contribute to the usefulness of SII in identifying patients that are more likely to experience severe infections as cervicofacial phlegmons. The only cells in the body that are capable of precisely identifying and detecting various antigens are lymphocytes. They are essential in the majority of chronic inflammatory lesions, particularly in autoimmune disorders and conditions with long-lasting antigens. The most crucial cellular defense against infections is provided by neutrophils, while platelets aid in hemostasis, inflammation, and host defense. With this in mind, SII is able to assess the equilibrium of the host's inflammatory and immunological condition.

The efficiency of this new index was demonstrated in case of patients diagnosed with cervicofacial phlegmons and other severe odontogenic infections. At the hospital admission of the cases, the calculated SII showed elevated levels that could be correlated with the poor general immune status of the patients. After the surgical treatment of the cervicofacial phlegmons was performed associated with the pharmacological treatment-antibiotherapy, AINS, the SII values decreased significantly [32, 33].

6.2 Neutrophil-Lymphocyte ratio (NLR)

Neutrophil and lymphocyte values are very important for assessing the evolution of cervicofacial phlegmons and for establishing a good prognosis of the cases. A typical reaction to the infectious process of the leucocytes is the increasing values in neutrophils. Compared to other WBC subpopulations, the neutrophil–lymphocyte ratio has a higher sensitivity in detecting the expansion of a systemic infection, being a useful biomarker for sepsis [34].

The NLR formula used for calculation is made by dividing the number of neutrophils by the number of lymphocytes. A normal range of NLR is between 1 and 2. The higher values 3 or smaller than 0.7 in adults are pathological (**Figure 4**) [35].

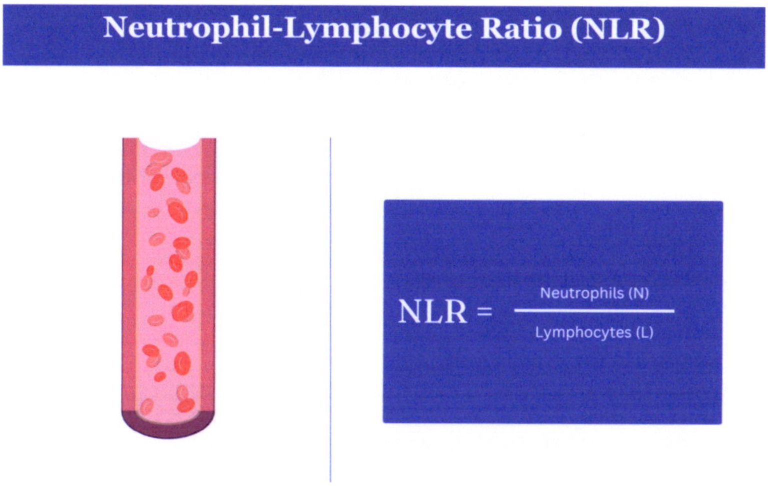

Figure 4.
The NLR formula (personal design and propriety of the authors).

The neutrophils involved in the phagocytosis process, which neutralizes the germs involved in the pathogeny of the cervicofacial phlegmons, are activated during the host response to a bacterial infection. Studies show that NLR levels rise in patients with deep neck infections, indicating that it may be a reliable indicator of bacteremia and sepsis.

Assessment of the NLR is a simple, easy, and cost-effective test for the quantification of the inflammatory status and complication risk in the case of neck infections. The NLR values are higher at hospital admission of patients with cervicofacial phlegmons. After a well-conducted surgical treatment of the cervicofacial phlegmons associated with the pharmacological treatment-antibiotherapy, AINS, the NLR values decreased significantly [32].

7. Conclusions

Systemic immune-inflammatory response plays a key role in the cervicofacial phlegmons' persistence, progression, and aggressiveness. A continuous monitorization of the relevant values of specific blood constituents that are strongly related to the individual response of the host could be the future approach for the management of these types of infections. Calculating and integrating from the beginning the systemic immune-inflammatory index and the presence of other inflammatory biomarkers and their response to the treatment offers a better prognosis for these cases.

Conflict of interest

The authors declare no conflict of interest.

Author details

Ciprian Ioan Roi[1], Alexandra Roi[2]* and Mircea Riviș[1]

1 Department of Anesthesiology and Oral Surgery, "Victor Babeș" University of Medicine and Pharmacy, Timișoara, Romania

2 Department of Oral Pathology, "Victor Babeș" University of Medicine and Pharmacy, Timișoara, Romania

*Address all correspondence to: alexandra.moga@umft.ro

References

[1] Bortnik P, Wieczorek P, Załęski P, Kosierkiewicz P, Siemiątkowski A, Tryniszewska E, et al. Odontogenic phlegmon of the mouth floor: A case report. Prog Health Sci. 2016;**6**(2):178-183

[2] Srirompotong S, Art-Smart T. Ludwig's angina: A clinical review. European Archives of Oto-Rhino-Laryngology. 2003;**260**(7):401-403. DOI: 10.1007/s00405-003-0588-9

[3] Bridwell R, Gottlieb M, Koyfman A, Long B. Diagnosis and management of Ludwig's angina: An evidence-based review. The American Journal of Emergency Medicine. 2021;**41**:1-5. DOI: 10.1016/j.ajem.2020.12.030

[4] Yamaguchi R, Sakurada K, Saitoh H, et al. Fatal airway obstruction due to Ludwig's angina from severe odontogenic infection during antipsychotic medication: A case report and a literature review. Journal of Forensic Sciences. 2021;**66**(5):1980-1985. DOI: 10.1111/1556-4029.14740

[5] Shemesh A, Yitzhak A, Ben Itzhak J, Azizi H, Solomonov M. Ludwig angina after first aid treatment: Possible Etiologies and prevention-case report. Journal of Endodontia. 2019;**45**(1):79-82. DOI: 10.1016/j.joen.2018.10.001

[6] Dowdy RAE, Emam HA, Cornelius BW. Ludwig's angina: Anesthetic management. Anesthesia Progress. 2019;**66**(2):103-110. DOI: 10.2344/anpr-66-01-13

[7] Levco S, Scerbatiuc D. Phlegmon of the oral floor. Contradictions in diagnosis and treatment. Mold. Medizinhistorisches Journal. 2018;**61**(1):42-48

[8] Uluibau IC, Jaunay T, Goss AN. Severe odontogenic infections. Australian Dental Journal. 2005;**50**(Suppl 2):S74-S81. DOI: 10.1111/j.1834 7819.2005.tb00390.x

[9] Hasegava J, Hidaka H, Tateda M. An analysis of clinical risk factors of deep neck infection. Auris, Nasus, Larynx. 2011;**38**:101-107

[10] Yilmaz S, Bas B, Ozden B, Selcuk U, Cengel KS. Deep neck infection after molar extraction. Journal of Istanbul University Faculty of Dentistry. 2015;**49**(2):41-45

[11] Benhoummad O, Cherrabi K, Ofri NE, Mortaji Z, Fakiri ME. Ludwig's angina in a child: A case report and literature review. The Egyptian Journal of Otolaryngology. 2023;**39**:74

[12] Banerjee S, Pathan AS. A rare case report of Ludwig's angina: Early detection and prevention of airway catastrophe. International Journal of Medical Reviews and Case Reports. 2022;**6**(20):30-33. DOI: 10.5455/IJMRCR.172-1667403497

[13] Kataria G, Saxena A, Bhagat S, Singh B, Kaur M. Deep neck space infections: A study of 76 cases. Iranian Journal of Otorhinolaryngology. 2015;**27**(81):293-299 32

[14] Reynolds SC, Chow AW. Life-threatening infections of the Peripharyngeal and deep fascial spaces of the head and neck. Infectious Disease Clinics of North America. 2007;**21**(2):557-576. DOI: 10.1016/j.idc.2007.03.002

[15] Fontoura de Melo TA, Rücker T, Dias do Carmo MP, Duarte Irala LE,

Azevedo Salles A. Ludwig's angina: Diagnosis and treatment. RSBO Revista Sul-Brasileira de Odontologia [Internet]. 2013;**10**(2):172-175. Recuperado de: https://www.redalyc.org/articulo.oa?id=153027495012

[16] Sakarozi R, Susilo DH. The use of neutrophil—Lymphocyte ratio (NLR) as a potential biomarker to predict the prognosis of Ludwig's angina patients. Bali Medical Journal. 2022;**11**:1553-1558. DOI: 10.15562/bmj.v11i3.3612

[17] Gordon NC, Connelly S. Management of head and neck infections in the immunocompromised patient. Oral and Maxillofacial Surgery Clinics of North America. 2003;**15**(1):103-110. DOI: 10.1016/s1042-3699(02)00079-1

[18] Rich R, Fleisher T, Schwartz B. Clincial Immunology and Practice. 3rd ed. St. Louis: Mosby-Year Book Inc; 2008

[19] Ortiz R, Espinoza V. Odontogenic infection. Review of the pathogenesis, diagnosis, complications and treatment. Res rep. Oral and Maxillofacial Surgery. 2021;**5**:055. DOI: 10.23937/2643-3907/1710055

[20] Kabanova AA, Pokhoden'ko–Chudakova IO, Kabanova SA. Systemic inflammatory response syndrome and serum Procalcitonin in odontogenic maxillofacial infection. I. P. Pavlov Russian Medical Biological Herald. 2023;**31**(1):119-125. DOI: 10.17816/PAVLOVJ106281

[21] Bali RK, Sharma P, Gaba S, Kaur A, Ghanghas P. A review of complications of odontogenic infections. National Journal of Maxillofacial Surgery. 2015;**6**:136-143

[22] Kusumoto J, Iwata E, Huang W, Takata N, Tachibana A, Akashi M. Hematologic and inflammatory parameters for determining severity of odontogenic infections at admission: A retrospective study. BMC Infectious Diseases. 2022;**22**(1):931. Published 2022 Dec 12. DOI: 10.1186/s12879-022-07934-x

[23] Pepys MB, Hirschfeld GM. C-reactive protein: a critical update. The Journal of Clinical Investigation. 2003;**111**:1805-1812

[24] Stathopoulos P, Igoumenakis D, Shuttleworth J, Smith W, Ameerally P. Predictive factors of hospital stay in patients with odontogenic maxillofacial infections: The role of C-reactive protein. The British Journal of Oral & Maxillofacial Surgery. 2017;**55**:367-370

[25] Sato FR, Hajala FA, Freire Filho FW, Moreira RW, de Moraes M. Eight-year retrospective study of odontogenic origin infections in a postgraduation program on oral and maxillofacial surgery. Journal of Oral and Maxillofacial Surgery. 2009;**67**(5):1092-1097. DOI: 10.1016/j.joms.2008.09.008

[26] Uppada UK, Sinha R. Outcome of odontogenic infections in rural setup: Our experience in management. Journal of Maxillofacial and Oral Surgery. 2020;**19**(1):113-118. DOI: 10.1007/s12663-019-01232-x

[27] Kim J.-K., Lee J.-H. Clinical utility of procalcitonin in severe odontogenic maxillofacial infection. Maxillofacial Plastic and Reconstructive Surgery. 2021. Vol. 43, № 1. P. 3. DOI: 10.1186/s40902-020-00288-x

[28] Wiedermann FJ, Kaneider N, Egger P, et al. Migration of human monocytes in response to procalcitonin. Critical Care Medicine. 2002;**30**(5):1112-1117

[29] Kang ES, Lee JH. Diagnostic value of presepsin in odontogenic infection: A retrospective study. Maxillofacial Plastic

and Reconstructive Surgery. 2022;**44**:22. DOI: 10.1186/s40902-022-00353-7

[30] Russell CD, Parajuli A, Gale HJ, et al. The utility of peripheral blood leucocyte ratios as biomarkers in infectious diseases: A systematic review and meta-analysis. The Journal of Infection. 2019;**78**(5):339-348. DOI: 10.1016/j.jinf.2019.02.006

[31] Liu X, Guan G, Cui X, Liu Y, Liu Y, Luo F. Systemic immune-inflammation index (SII) can Be an early indicator for predicting the severity of acute pancreatitis: A retrospective study. International Journal of General Medicine. 2021;**14**:9483-9489. Published 2021 Dec 8. DOI: 10.2147/IJGM.S343110

[32] Roi CI, Roi A, Nicoară A, Rivis m. Impact of treatment on systemic immune-inflammatory index and other inflammatory markers in odontogenic Cervicofacial Phlegmon cases: A retrospective study. Biomedicine. 2023;**11**(6):1710. Published 2023 Jun 14. DOI: 10.3390/biomedicines11061710

[33] Pricop M, Ancusa O, Talpos S, Urechescu H, Bumbu BA. The predictive value of systemic immune-inflammation index and symptom severity score for sepsis and systemic inflammatory response syndrome in odontogenic infections. Journal of Personalized Medicine. 2022;**12**(12):2026. Published 2022 Dec 7. DOI: 10.3390/jpm12122026

[34] Martins EC, Silveira LDF, Viegas K, et al. Neutrophil-lymphocyte ratio in the early diagnosis of sepsis in an intensive care unit: a case-control study. Razão neutrófilo-linfócito no diagnóstico precoce de sepse em unidade de terapia intensiva: um estudo de caso-controle. Revista Brasileira de Terapia Intensiva. 2019;**31**(1):64-70. DOI: 10.5935/0103-507X.20190010

[35] Baglam T, Binnetoglu A, Yumusakhuylu AC, Gerin F, Demir B, Sari M. Predictive value of the neutrophil-to-lymphocyte ratio in patients with deep neck space infection secondary to acute bacterial tonsillitis. International Journal of Pediatric Otorhinolaryngology. 2015;**79**(9):1421-1424. DOI: 10.1016/j.ijporl.2015.06.016

Chapter 5

Influence of Chronic Low-Grade Inflammation (Obesity) on the Systemic Inflammatory Response

Luz-Ma.-Adriana Balderas-Peña, Daniel Sat-Muñoz, Mario-Alberto Mireles-Ramírez, Brenda-Eugenia Martínez-Herrera, Arnulfo-Hernán Nava-Zavala, Luz-María Cervantes-González, Michelle-Guadalupe Muñoz-García, Benjamín Rubio-Jurado, Mario Salazar Páramo, Eduardo Gómez Sánchez and Carlos-M Nuño-Guzmán

Abstract

The chronic inflammatory state is a common condition in obesity. It has become a health problem with pandemic proportions that, in some developing countries, jointly to overweight, affects more than 50% of their population. As a part of the scenario, we observe how a significant proportion of people with overweight or obesity have raised the acute inflammatory response markers. This situation shows us how this chronic condition can trigger aggressive inflammatory phenomena in critically ill patients with other clinical conditions, occasioning torpid clinical evolution, ominous results, and low-rate survival. This chapter pretends to describe the influence of a low-grade inflammatory state on the clinical outcome of patients who develop a systemic inflammatory response.

Keywords: chronic diseases, low-rate inflammation, obesity, cancer, systemic inflammatory response

1. Introduction

The term inflammation has been known for over a thousand years, becoming the common pathway for different diseases [1]. In this way, inflammation becomes one of the essential physiological mechanisms of systemic regulation, a process where cellular and molecular events occur, decreasing injury progression, and restoring tissue homeostasis [2].

Homeostatic compensations, which are responses of organisms to damage, illness, or significant environmental challenges, can represent trade-offs required to preserve essential bodily processes but, over time, lead to further abnormalities in body function [3]. The immune system provides a mechanism for the body to discern between healthy foreign cells and substances and to phagocytose or produce sensitized lymphocytes, specialized proteins, or antibodies to eradicate the invader [3, 4]. When tissue suffers damage, the affected components yield several chemical substances, which significantly alter the proximity of healthy tissues. Therefore, inflammation refers to a complete range of tissue changes [3].

A natural conserved process in inflammation, regardless of being systemic or local, is defined by the activation of immune and non-immune cells that defend the host by removing cell damage, dropped, or altered host molecules (pathogens or endogenous), as well as toxins, while promoting tissue repair and recovery [5].

Evidence indicates how changes in metabolic and inflammatory processes affect several chemical compounds in the body [6]. The presence of inflammation plays a significant role as an indicator of complications or development of diseases such as overweight, obesity, diabetes mellitus, cardiovascular diseases, and cancer [7]. The excess fatty tissue produces a state of low-grade inflammation, and the presence of inflammatory markers establishes several links with pathways in some organs that can drive obesity-related inflammation [7].

Obesity worldwide is defined as excess adipose tissue [3]. The measure of body mass index (BMI), which is determined as follows, is a proxy indicator for body fat composition calculated by dividing the body weight in kilograms (kg) by the height squared (m^2); obesity is defined as BMI $\geq$ 30 kg/m^2 while overweight considered as BMI $\geq$25.0 kg/m^2 [3, 8, 9]; however, nowadays, it is recognized that BMI is a good screening tool, but it does not permit knowing the actual estimation of the fat mass and its impacts, such as the source of inflammatory mediators and endocrine organ; and ideally must be complemented by the body composition analysis, through different tools [DEXA (dual-energy X-ray absorptiometry), IMR (magnetic resonance imaging), BIA (bioelectrical impedance analysis), and themselves could be the objective of another discussion panel].

Nowadays, obesity has a 39% worldwide prevalence registered in 2021, existing strong evidence to support its close relationship to chronic low-grade systemic inflammation. The overweight obesity trendline considers the phenomenon one of the most important preventable risk factors for developing various chronic diseases [10], and it is linked to low-grade inflammatory phenomena.

During the COVID-19 pandemic, chronic low-grade inflammation was a common condition in patients with a severe hyperinflammatory syndrome, now named multisystemic inflammatory syndrome, defined by the centers for disease control and prevention (CDC) as a serious condition characterized by the presence of fever in a period over 24 hours, high levels of inflammatory markers and physical and biochemical evidence of multiorgan damage in a critically ill subject [11].

This chapter supports that this persistent medical condition can induce aggressive inflammatory processes (i.e., cytokine storm) in critically ill patients with diverse clinical disorders, leading to a sluggish clinical course, troubling outcomes, and a poor survival rate. This chapter explains how a low-grade inflammatory state impacts the patient's prognosis and offers an overview of the most severe disorders affecting the public's health worldwide.

2. Obesity and inflammatory phenomena impaction on intermediate metabolism

Overweight-obesity phenomenon is an altered metabolic condition and affects people at the pandemic global level; its origin is explained by a disproportionated relationship between energy intake and metabolic necessities and energy expenditure, and the result is the excess of adipose tissue (fat mass) that triggers a chronic low-grade inflammatory state.

A biological reaction to cellular damage, "inflammation," is characterized by interactions that predict disruption of immune homeostasis [12].

The inflammatory mechanisms are the expression of a nonspecific inflammatory response to any disruptor of the homeostasis in a biological organism and imply the activation of humoral and cellular mediators, such as the infiltrating macrophages located in the middle of the adipose tissue in a complex immunologic net of phenomena and triggering insulin resistance obesity-related [12].

As part of these complex inflammatory phenomena in the adipose tissue, various macrophage phenotypes lead to those cells' pro-inflammatory, anti-inflammatory, and even pleiotropic functions.

The immune system cell interacts with hypertrophic adipocytes through crosstalk, with chemotactic mediators that conduct the macrophage movements in infiltrating tissues, and consequently, the secretion of pro-inflammatory substances (TNFα, IL-6, IL-1 beta, and MCP-1, among others) and a chronic inflammatory state [13]. Monocyte–macrophages, described in 1882, are part of the innate immune system and represent one of the most primitive and unspecific host defense mechanisms in front of foreign pathogens, allergens, toxins, and even xenobiotic substances [12]. One of their most important roles is clearing cells and tissue damage, free chemotactic mediators, activating and solving sterile inflammatory events, and being the initial step for wound healing, tissue regeneration, and scar formation [13].

The molecules functioning, such as modulators for inflammation, depends on a broad group based on pattern recognition receptor, including toll-like receptors (TLRs), C-type lectin receptors (CLRs), nucleotide-binding oligomerization domain (NOD)-like receptors (NLRs), retinoic acid-inducible gene I (RIG-I)-like helicase receptors (RLR's), and scavenger receptors, among others [14]. Monocyte–macrophage identify more than 1000 molecular patterns, damage-associated and pathogen-associated (DAMP's and PAMP's), acting as immune mediators with a pleiotropic and dynamic profile of secreting products (cytokines, chemokines, and growth factors) [15].

The role of a chronic sterile inflammatory phenomenon has been better understood over the years and has been elucidated in areas such as allergy, autoimmune phenomena, and cancer, and a prominent clue position the interactive role of macrophages-adipose tissue during the insulin resistance obesity-induced and their satellite mechanisms [16–21].

Adipose tissue, functionally classified as white and brown adipose tissue (WAT and BAT, respectively), has a variety of metabolic actions. WAT goes 5 to 50% of total body weight; it is in subcutaneous, visceral epicardial, and around blood vessels; on the other hand, BAT has an inversely proportional relationship with age [22, 23]. The beige adipose tissue plays a heterogeneous role in glucose and lipid metabolism, helping to improve the intermediate metabolism [23].

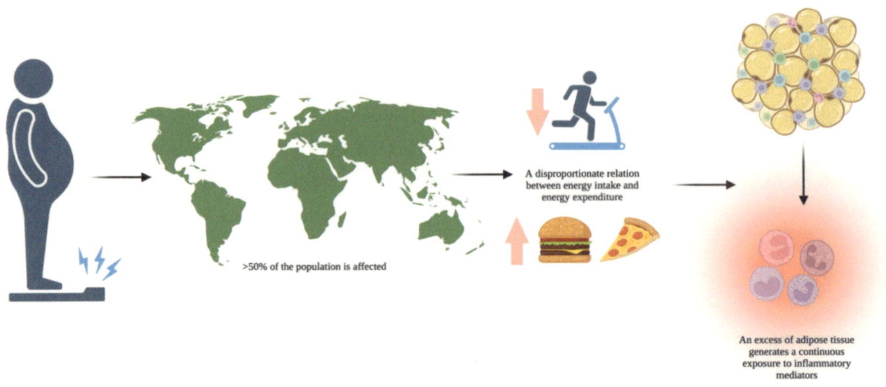

Figure 1.
Obesity and chronic inflammation. Obesity is one of the most prevalent diseases, affecting more than 50% of the population. This illness is explained by a disproportionated relation between energy intake and energy expenditure, which results in excess adipose tissue (considered an endocrine organ with chemotactic capabilities to produce endocrine signals from white adipose tissue) and puts patients into continuous exposure to inflammatory mediators, ending in a chronic inflammatory state that has diverse repercussions.

The homeostasis maintaining the adipose tissue is considered an endocrine organ, with chemotactic capabilities to produce endocrine signals from WAT [24]. In obese people, its functionally turns anomalous and expresses an inflammatory phenotype linked to systemic inflammation, metabolic syndrome, and insulin resistance [22]; in the whole process, TNFα is fundamental to the development of an inflammatory phenotype, besides TLR4 that is a crucial mediator molecule expressed in adipocytes and macrophages, involved in the induction of insulin resistance through fatty acids [25, 26] (**Figure 1**).

3. Inflammatory conditions on chronic diseases and their relationship with obesity

Chronic low-grade inflammation is joint in numerous chronic pathologies, some of which coincidentally have obesity according to the BMI of patients. Still, we know that it is not necessarily the better indicator of the quantity of fatty tissue in our body, and it is a good reason because currently is increasing the use of diverse tools to evaluate body composition in areas with a high prevalence of obesity.

The newest tools to determine the amount of fatty tissue overall and percentage involve all of them than discriminate lean mass, water, and fat mass such as IMR, computed tomography, and BIA. In the clinical ambulatory set, BIA has an advantage concerning IMR and CT and is a cost-effective tool that gives us information about subrogate measurements, such as phase angle, and has a predictive role in the patient outcome.

Fat mass is a source of lipids, an endocrine and metabolically active organ. Lipids forming the fat mass are involved in the innate immune response, specifically in triggering inflammatory mediators associated with the humoral immune unspecific response.

As we mentioned above, humoral inflammatory mediators are closely related to pleiotropic macrophage functions involved in various chronic conditions (coronary artery disease, diabetes type 2 obesity-related, or systemic unspecific response to damage in critically ill patients' ability to overcome or over-response with an acute inflammatory response [27].

Inflammatory processes are highly ontogenically conserved response physiological mechanisms. It has passed in an evolutive way, probably from an innate response to microbial inversion to an unspecific response to tissular damage in front of any damage mechanism [27].

It is one of the most ancient pathological processes recorded during human history; even classical Greeks *Celsus* and Galen described its cardinal signs: *rubber, heat, pain, tumor*, and loss of functioning [28].

The loss of control of the inflammation leads to damage in the systemic innate immune response, taking it to an imbalance between pro-, and anti-inflammatory molecular mediators, involving lipids, lysoglycerophospholipids, endocannabinoids, and their anatomical sources in the body. They all present in chronic disease development, such as cancer, diabetes mellitus, atherosclerosis, autoimmune diseases, and neurodegenerative processes, among other chronic inflammatory pathologies, which disrupt the tissular and systemic homeostasis [28].

The acute inflammatory response is triggered by innate immune cells such as macrophages, mast cells, and dendritic cells, involved in pathogen recognition through PAMPs or cell damage with impact on damage-associated molecular patterns (DAMPs). The complete cycle primarily induces local vasodilatation and cell recruitment, the release of complement proteins to stop microbes or molecules that have exceeded the epithelial or other natural barriers [28].

At this stage, the milieu has inflammatory characteristics with massive quantities of pro-inflammatory cytokines and omega-six-like pro-inflammatory lipid molecules as arachidonic acid-derived eicosanoids (prostaglandins and leukotrienes), all together potentiating the acute inflammatory immune response [29].

If the damage mechanisms stop the immune system and vascular endothelium put in on a lipid mediator class switch to break the eicosanoids and other inflammatory mediators, re-toward the metabolism to produce omega-three polyunsaturated fatty acids that initiate and lead the inflammatory phenomena to be solved. If the inflammation is extensive, it can be self-maintenance and promote the development of fibrosis and loss of tissular and organic functioning [30].

The acute inflammatory processes can be perpetuated secondary to the persistence of the damage source or *via* an abnormal and exaggerated inflammatory response, and then the acute inflammation turns into a chronic process, where the imbalance between pro-inflammatory and anti-inflammatory cytokines is disrupted. Bioactive lipids and fatty tissue have a predominant role in the continuous recruitment of immune cells such as macrophages, effector T helper lymphocytes, B cells, and T regulatory cells as part of an uncontrolled immune inflammatory response joined to abnormal tissue remodeling, irreversible and chronic tissue damage, and disease symptoms. The chronic inflammatory response is bounded to most human diseases (cancer, autoimmune diseases, metabolic alterations, cardiovascular diseases, and neurodegenerative processes) [31, 32] (**Figure 2**).

3.1 Inflammation and diabetes

Diabetes is one of the more prevalent chronic diseases around the world, and type 2 is usually associated with the complex overweight-obesity and insulin resistance; all of them involved in an imbalance between energy intake and expenditure, with the accumulation of fat mass and the consequent chronic low-grade inflammatory state,

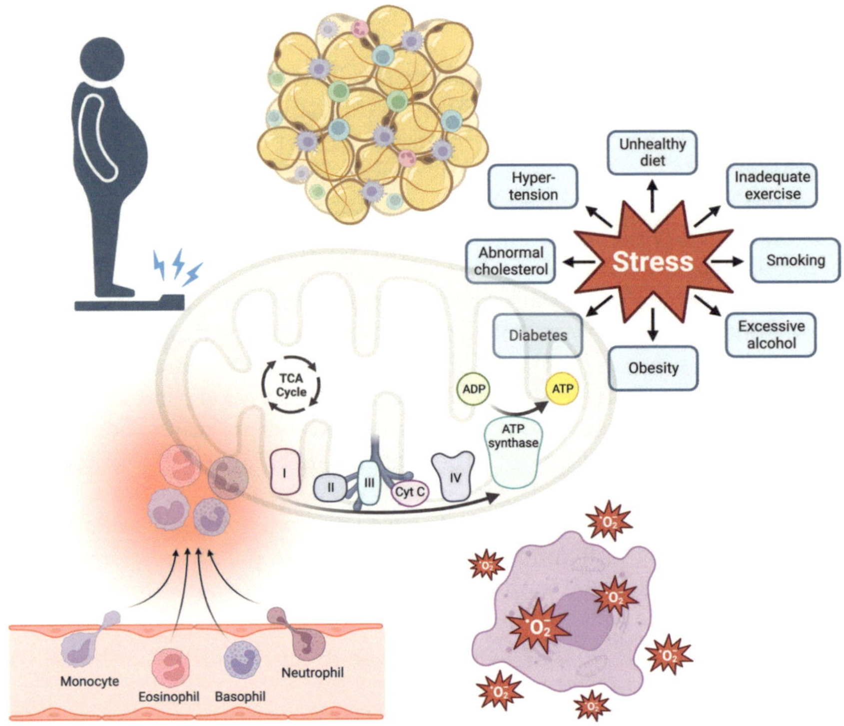

Figure 2.
Chronic low-grade inflammation and chronic diseases. Chronic low-grade inflammation is joint in numerous chronic pathologies, some of which coincidentally have obesity, where the immune system cell plays a fundamental role in interacting with hypertrophic adipocytes through crosstalk, with chemotactic mediators that conduct the macrophage movements in infiltrating tissues, and consequently, the secretion of pro-inflammatory substances (TNFα, IL-6, IL-1 beta, MCP-1, among others).

with macrophage activation through chemotactic signals from high-lipid content adipocytes, and consequently, elevated levels of pro-inflammatory cytokines that perpetuate the insulin resistance in obesity. It predisposes to the development of diabetes mellitus type 2 [13, 33].

The effects of the adipose tissue are endothelial dysfunction and the subsequent development of cardiovascular diseases. As a shred of evidence, in this milieu, a complex cross-talking between endocrine, immune (chronic inflammatory state), and neuronal networks is developing, relating to the loss of insulin sensitivity in target cells (adipocytes, hepatocytes, and myocytes immune cells, among others). This condition alters the insulin ability to control glucose levels and lipid homeostasis toward hyperglycemia, hyperlipidemia, and clinical data of diabetes type 2 [34, 35].

In the initial steps, the alterations are partially compensated through an increased insulin release and secretion from pancreatic beta-cells, leading to the exhaust of the beta-cells, reduced expression of insulin receptors, and altered metabolic feedback for the insulin [36, 37], perpetuating the chronic inflammatory state in the liver, skeletal muscle mass, endocrine pancreatic islets, and brain.

In the concrete case of obesity and inflammation related to metabolic diseases, the senescence of cells joins the aging to chronic disorders. Then aging enhances the burden of cellular senescence in almost all tissues with metabolic activity during the pathophysiological process of obesity in adulthood, diabetes mellitus type 2, and nonalcoholic fatty liver related to obesity, independently from the aging alone [38].

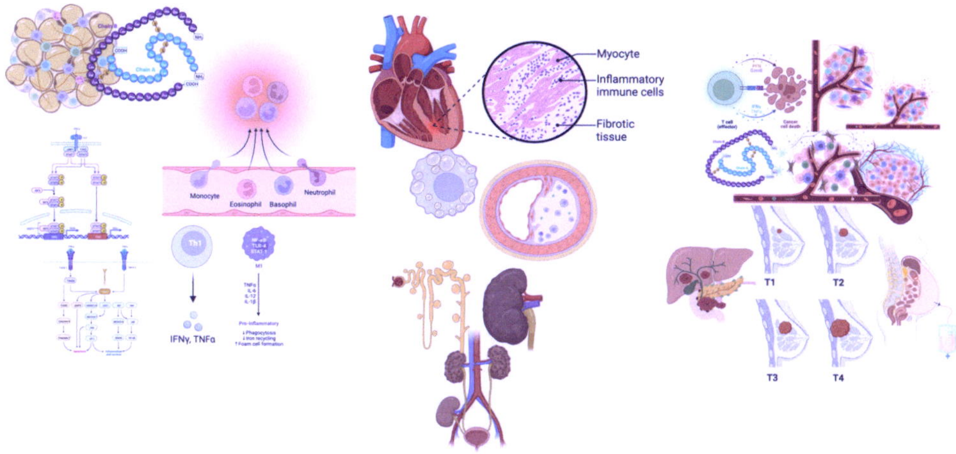

Figure 3.
Loss of control of inflammatory-anti-inflammatory balance and chronic diseases. The loss of control of inflammation leads to damage in the systemic innate immune response, taking it to an imbalance between pro, and anti-inflammatory molecular mediators, generating metabolic disturbances linked to low-grade chronic inflammation, promoting obesity-related hyperglycemia, insulin signaling, and high activity of glycolytic pathway and oxidative stress, reactions which end up triggering a low-grade chronic inflammatory state and being a central factor for many other diseases, as diabetes, cardiovascular diseases, chronic kidney disease, and even some types of cancer.

The senescence has a profound effect on the cells and toward the tissues to be dysfunctional and show inflammation stigmas in progenitor and mature cells, well-differentiated, or non-proliferating cells [38].

The insulin resistance-hyperinsulinemia pathophysiologic way, triggering senescence tissue in human adipose and liver cells, and the senescence perpetuate the insulin resistance in a vicious circle that profoundly affects people with these metabolic issues in age, body mass index, and hyperinsulinemia degree independent mechanism [39].

All the above-described phenomena reflect the relevance of the inflammatory mechanisms in obesity, insulin resistance, and diabetes and their profound effect on the health-disease interplay in humans (**Figure 3**).

3.2 Inflammation and cardiovascular diseases (hypertension, ischemic cardiopathy, and stroke)

In cardiovascular diseases, atherosclerosis is essential and involves molecular mechanisms that result reflected in pathophysiologic issues joined to an inflammatory response. Recent publications describe the pro-inflammatory cellular stress, the role of the endothelium, and its functioning releasing molecules with autocrine, paracrine, and endocrine actions that sequentially trigger and perpetuate the inflammatory low-grade phenomena in cardiovascular disease and stroke, which are characteristics of the immune response that lead to inflammation and turn an atheroma plaque stable to unstable [40].

Various mechanisms induce inflammatory processes in atherosclerosis, including endothelium aging, metabolism alterations, and autoimmune and infectious damage. Along the described mechanisms, atherosclerosis triggers life-threat pathophysiological conditions such as cardiogenic shock, myocardial infarction, and stroke, all of them with acute systemic hyperinflammation that potentiate other phenomena such as procoagulant cascades, coinciding both kinds of inflammatory processes acute and chronic [41].

Atherosclerosis represents an inflammatory disease with a chronicity trend, affecting the elastic and muscular line in the arterial vessels, implicating the formation of atheroma plaques (rich in cholesterol) that cause obstruction and stenosis in the stable plaque and thrombosis in unstable plaque due to the activation of complement and coagulation cascades [40].

Regarding atherosclerosis pathophysiology, the inflammation that characterizes the disease is joined to aging but is not necessarily the only factor; it could be related to obesity, insulin resistance with cellular senescence, and genetic predisposition (familial dyslipidemias), among others [42]. The inflammatory phenomenon can be considered as nonclassical inflammation (**Figure 3**).

3.3 Chronic kidney disease and inflammation

Chronic kidney disease has become one of the most common illnesses worldwide, especially in low- and middle-income countries, reaching over 800 million people globally with this diagnosis (10% of the overall population) and emerging as one of the leading causes of mortality [43].

Persistent low-grade inflammation is an elemental factor in this disease's development, making the kidneys one of the most highly susceptible organs to damage from pro-inflammatory cytokines and oxidative stress [44]. The renal system controls a significant portion of blood circulation, with the kidneys as the primary organs for maintaining the corticomedullary osmotic gradient for fluid absorption and urine concentration [45].

In the face of stressors such as energy deprivation, hormones, and various vasoactive molecules (including prostaglandins and nitric oxide) are produced to maintain homeostasis. However, these regulatory molecules are disrupted when inflammation results in kidney damage [46].

Renal tubules also contain many inflammatory markers responsible for renal insults and damage. Nevertheless, in remark to dysregulation states, such as diabetes, complications of acute kidney injury, and other uncontrolled inflammatory responses, these inflammatory mediators stop being regulated, which contributes to maladaptive response, higher energy demands, and a significant risk to ischemia, leading to oxidative damage as well, secondary to increased reactive oxygen species and decreased nitric oxide due to increased homocysteine levels [47].

Other factors trigger the emergence of a constant inflammation cascade that involves the patients with this diagnosis, which, in addition to the previous mechanism, occurs as a result of the treatment that has been given, for example, in dialysis, where factors such as impurities, microorganism presence, and even genetic and epigenetic influence, make the patient prone to an increase in the production of pro-inflammatory cytokines and oxidative stress, contributing to chronic inflammatory status [48].

CKD, then, is linked to an inflammatory state, and some authors describe the role of low-grade systemic inflammation in the development of CKD with alterations in laboratory inflammatory markers frequently coincidental with metabolic syndrome, nonalcoholic fatty liver disease, diabetes type 2, or cardiovascular disease [45, 48, 49]. As in other pathological conditions, the inflammatory phenomenon initiates with pro-inflammatory cytokines release, with an increased blood flow and chemotaxis mediating leukocyte infiltration [50]. The inflammatory low-grade state persists and is perpetuated by phenomena such as poor diet, alterations in gut microbiota, pregnancy in women, childhood infections, and cell stress in a previous phase of the disease establishment [51].

In CKD, substantial settings enhance and perpetuate the inflammatory state, infections, malnourishment, oxidative stress, dyslipidemia, overload volume, dialysis, and reduced clearance of inflammatory mediators [44].

The kidneys are essential to maintaining homeostasis, along they are involved with clearing cytokines and foreign antigens during renal clearance, removing pro-inflammatory cytokines and PAMPs as part of the kidney mechanisms that control the inflammation [51]. The tissue kidney interaction with renal dendritic cells and macrophages subtype M2 generates immune tolerance phenomena.

The own renal mechanism limits the inflammatory processes. It helps to immune tolerance, causing high susceptibility to damage mediated by inflammatory molecules in the kidney, which receives approximately 25% of the cardiac output in a minute, turning over to the kidney propensity to damage by inflammation and chronic renal damage, exacerbated by endothelial compromise by ischemic phenomena [52, 53] (**Figure 3**).

3.4 Cancer and inflammation

Adipose tissue is dysfunctional in obesity and even in overweight. The crosstalk between microenvironmental conditions, adipocytes, and immune system cells turns the typical phenotype of the cells to a malignant phenotype characterized by immortal cells with loss of mechanisms that control the proliferation in an altered context of endocrine signals that promote cancer development through autocrine, paracrine, and endocrine cell signaling [11].

In 2016, after analyzing over 1000 epidemiological reports, the IARC Working Group published a viewpoint [54]. Enough evidence exists to conclude that obesity is related to cancer development in at least thirteen anatomical locations, with a broad spectrum of pathophysiologic alterations in association with overweight-obesity and their involvement from sex hormone metabolism to intermediate metabolism disturbances (e.g., insulin resistance), adipocytokine expression with an exacerbated pro-inflammatory-oxidative status [55–57].

As part of the metabolic alterations in obesity, adipocytes have subcellular and metabolic disturbances that include endoplasmic reticulum and mitochondrial dysfunction, with an enhanced level of reactive oxygen species as a direct consequence of an overload of nutrients, conditions that generate a microenvironment favoring the inflammation, metabolic disturbance (dyslipidemia, hyperglycemia, and oxidative stress) inducing DNA damage and genomic instability, linked to low-grade chronic inflammation, joined to obesity-related hyperglycemia, enhanced insulin signaling, high activity of glycolytic pathway, and oxidative stress [57–65].

All previously mentioned changes influence the relationship between cell–cell and cell-extracellular matrix in tumors located in the vicinity of areas with adipose tissue [65], with a variety of common pathways with mechanisms involved with chronic low-grade inflammatory phenomena and all together promote angiogenesis, invasion, metalloproteinase activation, reactive oxygen species release mediated through molecular ways such as phosphoinositide 3-kinase (PI3K), vascular endothelial growth factor (VEGF), and signaling interplay such as PI3K/Akt [66–72].

To sum up, in cancer, one of the most critical elements to condition the tissue malignant transformation is obesity and its influence on the chronic or sustained low-grade inflammation with metabolic disruption, elevated tissue levels of pro-inflammatory cytokines, C reactive protein, and others that reinforce the pro-inflammatory context generating a deleterious effect on the nutritional state of cancer patients increasing the malnourishment related to tumor-cachexia and significant inflammatory mediators levels [73].

Then cancer occurs by chronic inflammatory pathway activation and a failure to resolve them [74]. In this scenario, the substantial effect of the molecular mechanisms that induce obesity generates a relationship in carcinogenesis [74]. The elevated levels of pro-inflammatory molecules make a microenvironment disrupt cell processes [75]. Inflammation in obese produces a dysregulated innate immunity activation of cytokines in adipocytokine metabolism, potentially enhancing angiogenesis and tumor progression [74]. The mechanisms identify with the prolonged inflammation that contributes to the proliferation of cancer with angiogenesis, tissue remodeling, and DNA damage [75]. A mechanism identifier is in the regulation of p53 (tumor suppressor gene). The evidence shows that chronic levels of inflammation in tumorigenicity can result from the inhibition of this gene with the inhibited cell apoptosis induced in cell proliferation [75]. The presence of increased levels in inflammation parameters (interleukin IL-1, IL-6, and C–reactive protein) and oxidative stress (glutathione peroxidase and superoxide dismutase) contributes to the cell damage that promotes the development of types of cancer such as breast, colorectal, esophageal, and liver cancer [76].

Cancer has a close relationship with obesity, and obesity exerts a profound influence on insulin resistance, arterial hypertension, dyslipidemia, and other disturbances in the intermediate metabolism. During the rapid increase of the obesity pandemic, cancer cases rose too, and then began the explosion of papers describing

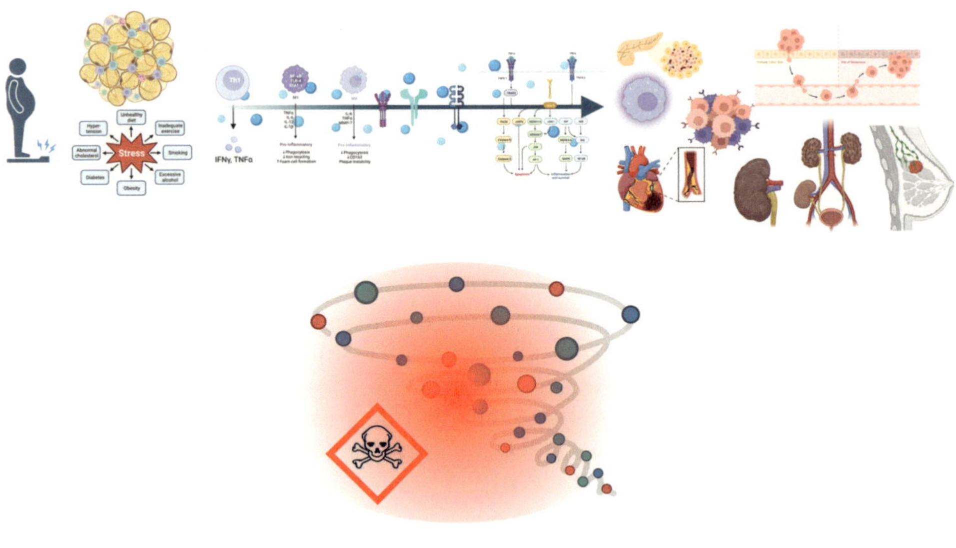

Figure 4.
Resumé low-grade chronic inflammation associated with chronic diseases and Acute Hyperinflammation. As part of the metabolic alterations in obesity, adipocytes have subcellular and metabolic disturbances that include endoplasmic reticulum and mitochondrial dysfunction, with an enhanced level of reactive oxygen species as a direct consequence of an overload of nutrients, conditions that generate a microenvironment favoring the inflammation, metabolic disturbance (dyslipidemia, hyperglycemia, and oxidative stress) inducing DNA damage, and genomic instability.

the influence of obesity and low-grade inflammation in the genesis, maintenance, and progression of various malignant diseases [77]. The interplay between adipose tissue, immune system cells, and molecules and the development of malignant cells reflect a homeostatic disruption in the balance between the anti-inflammatory and pro-inflammatory milieu [77].

In the case of cancer, macrophages play a crucial role in development and progression. Still, they are not the only involved cells B lymphocytes interact too in sustained inflammatory conditions [78]; besides pro-inflammatory mediators such as adipocytokines, that join to dyslipidemia, hyperglycemia, and hypercholesterolemia worsening the health biological behavior of the macrophages and potentiate their detrimental effects [78] (**Figures 3** and **4**).

4. Influence of chronic inflammatory conditions on the clinical outcomes in acute situations (acute systemic inflammatory response)

The presence of a chronic state with low-grade systemic inflammation plays an essential role in the etiology and pathogenesis of multiple diseases [79]. The evidence demonstrates a link between chronic inflammation and acute exacerbation in various illnesses [80]. Inflammatory cytokines such as IL-6 and tumor necrosis factor-alpha (TNF-alpha), created after persistent inflammation and oxidative stress, start a vicious cycle [80].

Despite the previously mentioned mechanisms, the chronic low-grade inflammatory state in aging diseases belongs to phenomena named nonclassical inflammation (meta-inflammation, quasi-inflammation, or para-inflammation) [28, 81–84], and it is part of an ontogenic mechanism evolutive preserved to the maintenance of homeostasis (allostasis; understanding as they achieve the stability through a changing milieu), and it involves the vascular endothelium, immune system, and lipid metabolism primarily in response to different challenges induced by the internal or external conditions [84].

In the tissues, the pro-inflammatory mechanisms include a feedback loop to synthesize and release mediators, such as cytokines, even in diseases not considered inflammatory states per se (cancer, neurologic, and psychiatric disorders) [85–88].

The term canonical inflammation has recently re-emerged. It is characterized by a focal reaction in the microvascular bed and triggers an exudative response with leukocyte migration by chemotaxis to the local damaged tissues. The pathophysiological mechanisms involve endothelial response at the level of postcapillary venules, causing endothelitis, a phenomenon observed only in vertebrates with lymphatic microcapillaries net and microcirculatory units in various organs. It generated the classical signs of inflammation (rubor (redness), tumor, heat, pain, and loss of function) [89, 90]. On the other hand, invertebrates develop nonclassical local inflammation, characterized by phagocyte accumulation in damaged tissue, without any microvascular compromise [89].

In any inflammatory process, the goal of the local inflammation is to isolate and eliminate any damage-related damage. Still, in the low-grade inflammatory response, the four local signs of inflammation are not involved in the sustained response [87, 89].

The low-grade inflammation is known as para-inflammation, and it is considered a nonclassical type of inflammation with long-term effects of the factors damage-related, in the absence of signs of an inflammatory focus, delocalization of the process, not enough mechanical barriers, interconnected with the tissular aging, metabolic mediators related to damage and systemic changes in the endothelium (endotheliosis; all of them observed in metabolic syndrome, morbid obesity, DM type 2, and aging-related sarcopenia) [91, 92].

Based on the inflammatory mechanisms previously named, recently has been delineated the hyperinflammation or high-grade systemic inflammatory state, tied to an exacerbated systemic effect of inflammation, triggers mediators leading to systemic endothelitis, resulting in life-threatening endothelial disorders, joined to leukocytes activation inside blood vessels, with subsequent activation of hemostatic mechanisms, complements factors and kallikrein-kinin systems.

In patients who have a basis of low-grade chronic inflammatory state related to obesity, metabolic alterations, and aging, among others, a new damage condition can release a cytokine storm, enhancing the latent microcirculatory issues, perpetuating the damage that could be limited in an acute inflammatory state, turning it severe and transforming in a life treating condition, such as in severe COVID-19 and the cytokine storm observed in obese and diabetic patients.

Therefore, the confluence of the local and systemic chronic-low-level inflammation and acute inflammatory conditions can lead to the perfect storm where the chronic conditions inflammation-related will worsen the inflammatory response in current damage and turn over the phenomena to hyperinflammation (**Figure 4**).

5. Conclusions

Chronic low-grade inflammatory state derived from obesity is a present condition in a wide variety of chronic and aging-related diseases, such as diabetes type 2, cardiovascular diseases and stroke, chronic kidney disease, and cancer, among the most important. During the past four years, we observed a "perfect storm" of the coincidental phenomena involving chronic low-grade inflammation in chronic diseases and emerging acute diseases with an exacerbating inflammatory response, clearly represented by severe COVID-19 cases [93], triggering a multisystemic inflammatory syndrome worsening the prognosis in critically ill patients. Throughout the process, we understood how the chronic low-grade inflammatory states allied to aging-related diseases potentiate the systemic acute response triggering a massive release of inflammatory mediators, generating the now-named "cytokine storm" and putting in this scenario the fundamental importance of regulating and modifying the people behavior to turn to a healthier lifestyle, reducing the overweight-obesity rates around the world through a better diet and increasing the rates of physical activity, to improve their health conditions and health-related quality of life through the changes in modifiable risk factors.

Conflict of interest

The authors declare no conflict of interest.

Author details

Luz-Ma.-Adriana Balderas-Peña[1*], Daniel Sat-Muñoz[2*],
Mario-Alberto Mireles-Ramírez[3], Brenda-Eugenia Martínez-Herrera[4],
Arnulfo-Hernán Nava-Zavala[5,7], Luz-María Cervantes-González[6],
Michelle-Guadalupe Muñoz-García[6], Benjamín Rubio-Jurado[8],
Mario Salazar Páramo[9], Eduardo Gómez Sánchez[10] and Carlos-M Nuño-Guzmán[11]

1 Biomedical Research Unit 02, UMAE Specialties Hospital National Western Medical Center, IMSS (from the Spanish: Instituto Mexicano del Seguro Social) and Morphology Department at the University of Guadalajara, Mexico

2 Oncologic Surgery Department, UMAE Specialties Hospital National Western Medical Center, IMSS (from the Spanish: Instituto Mexicano del Seguro Social) and Morphology Department at the University of Guadalajara, Mexico

3 Health Research Division, UMAE Specialties Hospital National Western Medical Center, IMSS, Mexico

4 Nutrition and Diet Department, General Zone Hospital #1. Órgano de Operación Administrativa Desconcentrada (OOAD) Estatal Aguascalientes, Instituto Mexicano del Seguro Social. Cd. Aguascalientes, Aguascalientes, México

5 Social, Epidemiologic, and Health Services Research Unit, OOAD State Jalisco, International Program, Medicine, Autonomous University of Guadalajara, Mexico

6 Biomedical Research Unit 02, UMAE Specialties Hospital National Western Medical Center, IMSS (from the Spanish: Instituto Mexicano del Seguro Social); Academic coordination of Medicine Career at the University of Guadalajara, Mexico, and fellow on General Direction on Health Quality and Education, Health Secretary, Mexico

7 Rheumatology and Immunology Service, Internal Medicine Division, Western General Hospital, Mexico

8 Hematology Clinical Department, UMAE Specialties Hospital National Western Medical Center, IMSS (from the Spanish: Instituto Mexicano del Seguro Social), Mexico

9 Physiology Department, Immunology Academy, University of Guadalajara, Mexico

10 Clinical Disciplines Division, University of Guadalajara, Mexico

11 Surgery Department, UMAE Specialties Hospital National Western Medical Center, IMSS (from the Spanish: Instituto Mexicano del Seguro Social) and Clinical Disciplines Division, University of Guadalajara, Mexico

*Address all correspondence to: luz.balderas@academicos.udg.mx and daniel.sat@academicos.udg.mx

References

[1] Medzhitov R. Inflammation 2010: New adventures of an old flame. Cell. 2010;**140**(6):771-776

[2] Chen L, Deng H, Cui H, Fang J, Zuo Z, Deng J, et al. Inflammatory responses and inflammation-associated diseases in organs. Oncotarget. 2018;**9**(6):7204-7218

[3] Hall JE, Hall ME. Tratado de fisiología médica. 14th ed. Barcelona: Elsevier; 2021

[4] Lemke G. How macrophages deal with death. Nature Reviews. Immunology. 2019;**19**(9):539-549

[5] Netea MG, Balkwill F, Chonchol M, Cominelli F, Donath MY, Giamarellos-Bourboulis EJ, et al. A guiding map for inflammation. Nature Immunology. 2017;**18**(8):826-831

[6] Rosen ED, Spiegelman BM. What we talk about when we talk about fat. Cell. 2014;**156**(1-2):20-44

[7] Lempesis IG, Georgakopoulou VE. Physiopathological mechanisms related to inflammation in obesity and type 2 diabetes mellitus. World Journal of Experimental Medicine. 2023;**13**(3):7-16

[8] Szukiewicz D. Molecular mechanisms for the vicious cycle between insulin resistance and the inflammatory response in obesity. IJMS. 2023;**24**(12):9818

[9] Cuciureanu M, Caratașu CC, Gabrielian L, Frăsinariu OE, Checheriță LE, Trandafir LM, et al. 360-degree perspectives on obesity. Medicina. 2023;**59**(6):1119

[10] Sanhueza S, Simón L, Cifuentes M, Quest AFG. The adipocyte–macrophage relationship in cancer: A potential target for antioxidant therapy. Antioxidants. 2023;**12**(1):126

[11] Hamad Saied M, van der Griend L, van Straalen JW, Wulffraat NM, Vastert S, Jansen MHA. The protective effect of COVID-19 vaccines on developing multisystem inflammatory syndrome in children (MIS-C): A systematic literature review and meta-analysis. Pediatric Rheumatology Online Journal. 2023;**21**(1):80

[12] Minihane AM, Vinoy S, Russell WR, Baka A, Roche HM, Tuohy KM, et al. Low-grade inflammation, diet composition and health: Current research evidence and its translation. The British Journal of Nutrition. 2015;**114**(7):999-1012

[13] Guria S, Hoory A, Das S, Chattopadhyay D, Mukherjee S. Adipose tissue macrophages and their role in obesity-associated insulin resistance: An overview of the complex dynamics at play. Bioscience Reports. 2023;**43**(3):BSR20220200

[14] Palm NW, Medzhitov R. Pattern recognition receptors and control of adaptive immunity. Immunological Reviews. 2009;**227**(1):221-233

[15] Zhang X, Mosser D. Macrophage activation by endogenous danger signals. The Journal of Pathology. 2008;**214**(2):161-178

[16] Sica A, Mantovani A. Macrophage plasticity and polarization: in vivo veritas. The Journal of Clinical Investigation. 2012;**122**(3):787-795

[17] Reese TA, Liang HE, Tager AM, Luster AD, Van Rooijen N, Voehringer D,

et al. Chitin induces accumulation in tissue of innate immune cells associated with allergy. Nature. 2007;**447**(7140):92-96

[18] Ma WT, Gao F, Gu K, Chen DK. The role of monocytes and macrophages in autoimmune diseases: A comprehensive review. Frontiers in Immunology. 2019;**10**:1140

[19] Qian BZ, Li J, Zhang H, Kitamura T, Zhang J, Campion LR, et al. CCL2 recruits inflammatory monocytes to facilitate breast-tumour metastasis. Nature. 2011;**475**(7355):222-225

[20] Weisberg SP, McCann D, Desai M, Rosenbaum M, Leibel RL, Ferrante AW. Obesity is associated with macrophage accumulation in adipose tissue. The Journal of Clinical Investigation. 2003;**112**(12):1796-1808

[21] Xu H, Barnes GT, Yang Q, Tan G, Yang D, Chou CJ, et al. Chronic inflammation in fat plays a crucial role in the development of obesity-related insulin resistance. The Journal of Clinical Investigation. 2003;**112**(12):1821-1830

[22] Chait A, Den Hartigh LJ. Adipose tissue distribution, inflammation and its metabolic consequences, including diabetes and cardiovascular disease. Frontier in Cardiovascular Medicine. 2020;**7**:22

[23] Li Y, Yun K, Mu R. A review on the biology and properties of adipose tissue macrophages involved in adipose tissue physiological and pathophysiological processes. Lipids in Health and Disease. 2020;**19**(1):164

[24] Kershaw EE, Flier JS. Adipose tissue as an endocrine organ. The Journal of Clinical Endocrinology & Metabolism. 2004;**89**(6):2548-2556

[25] Nisoli E, Briscini L, Giordano A, Tonello C, Wiesbrock SM, Uysal KT, et al. Tumor necrosis factor α mediates apoptosis of brown adipocytes and defective brown adipocyte function in obesity. Proceedings of the National Academic Science USA. 2000;**97**(14):8033-8038

[26] Shi H, Kokoeva MV, Inouye K, Tzameli I, Yin H, Flier JS. TLR4 links innate immunity and fatty acid–induced insulin resistance. The Journal of Clinical Investigation. 2006;**116**(11):3015-3025

[27] Radzioch D, Giera M, De Sanctis JB. Editorial: Quo Vadis lipid mediators – Lipid mediators implication in inflammation and chronic inflammatory diseases. Frontiers in Immunology. 2021;**12**:699276

[28] Medzhitov R. Origin and physiological roles of inflammation. Nature. 2008;**454**(7203):428-435

[29] Dennis EA, Norris PC. Eicosanoid storm in infection and inflammation. Nature Reviews. Immunology. 2015;**15**(8):511-523

[30] Levy BD, Clish CB, Schmidt B, Gronert K, Serhan CN. Lipid mediator class switching during acute inflammation: Signals in resolution. Nature Immunology. 2001;**2**(7):612-619

[31] Fullerton JN, Gilroy DW. Resolution of inflammation: A new therapeutic frontier. Nature Reviews. Drug Discovery. 2016;**15**(8):551-567

[32] Aoki T, Narumiya S. Prostaglandins and chronic inflammation. Trends in Pharmacological Sciences. 2012;**33**(6):304-311

[33] Harford KA, Reynolds CM, McGillicuddy FC, Roche HM. Fats, inflammation and insulin resistance: Insights to the role of macrophage and T-cell accumulation in adipose tissue.

The Proceedings of the Nutrition Society. 2011;**70**(4):408-417

[34] Engin AB. Adipocyte-macrophage cross-talk in obesity. In: Engin AB, Engin A, editors. Obesity and Lipotoxicity. Cham: Springer International Publishing; 2017. pp. 327-343. Available from: http://link.springer.com/10.1007/978-3-319-48382-5_14

[35] Asterholm IW, Halberg N, Scherer PE. Mouse models of lipodystrophy: Key reagents for the understanding of the metabolic syndrome. Drug Discovery Today: Disease Models. 2007;**4**(1):17-24

[36] Mukhuty A, Fouzder C, Mukherjee S, Malick C, Mukhopadhyay S, Bhattacharya S, et al. Palmitate induced Fetuin-A secretion from pancreatic β-cells adversely affects its function and elicits inflammation. Biochemical and Biophysical Research Communications. 2017;**491**(4):1118-1124

[37] Jia Q, Morgan-Bathke ME, Jensen MD. Adipose tissue macrophage burden, systemic inflammation, and insulin resistance. American Journal of Physiology-Endocrinology and Metabolism. 2020;**319**(2):E254-E264

[38] Gustafson B, Nerstedt A, Spinelli R, Beguinot F, Smith U. Type 2 diabetes, independent of obesity and age, is characterized by senescent and dysfunctional mature human adipose cells. Diabetes. 2022;**71**(11):2372-2383

[39] Spinelli R, Baboota RK, Gogg S, Beguinot F, Blüher M, Nerstedt A, et al. Increased cell senescence in human metabolic disorders. Journal of Clinical Investigation. 2023;**133**(12):e169922

[40] Gusev E, Sarapultsev A. Atherosclerosis and inflammation: Insights from the theory of general pathological processes. IJMS. 2023;**24**(9):7910

[41] Xiang Q, Tian F, Xu J, Du X, Zhang S, Liu L. New insight into dyslipidemia-induced cellular senescence in atherosclerosis. Biological Reviews. 2022;**97**(5):1844-1867

[42] Santos RD, Gidding SS, Hegele RA, Cuchel MA, Barter PJ, Watts GF, et al. Defining severe familial hypercholesterolaemia and the implications for clinical management: A consensus statement from the international atherosclerosis society severe familial hypercholesterolemia panel. The Lancet Diabetes & Endocrinology. 2016;**4**(10):850-861

[43] Kovesdy CP. Epidemiology of chronic kidney disease: An update 2022. Kidney International Supplements. 2022;**12**(1):7-11

[44] Kadatane SP, Satariano M, Massey M, Mongan K, Raina R. The role of inflammation in CKD. Cell. 2023;**12**(12):1581

[45] Mihai S, Codrici E, Popescu ID, Enciu AM, Albulescu L, Necula LG, et al. Inflammation-related mechanisms in chronic kidney disease prediction, progression, and outcome. Journal of Immunology Research. 2018;**2018**:1-16

[46] Damkjær M, Vafaee M, Møller ML, Braad PE, Petersen H, Høilund-Carlsen PF, et al. Renal cortical and medullary blood flow responses to altered NO availability in humans. American Journal of Physiology-Regulatory, Integrative and Comparative Physiology. 2010;**299**(6):R1449-R1455

[47] Liu BC, Tang TT, Lv LL, Lan HY. Renal tubule injury: A driving force toward chronic kidney disease. Kidney International. 2018;**93**(3):568-579

[48] Akchurin OM, Kaskel F. Update on inflammation in chronic kidney disease. Blood Purification. 2015;**39**(1-3):84-92

[49] United States Renal Data System. 2022 USRDS Annual Data Report: Epidemiology of Kidney Disease in the United States. National Institutes of Health; 2022

[50] Pahwa R, Goyal A, Jialal I. Chronic Inflammation. Treasure Island, FL: StatPearls Publishing; 2023. Available from: http://www.ncbi.nlm.nih.gov/books/NBK493173/

[51] Kurts C, Panzer U, Anders HJ, Rees AJ. The immune system and kidney disease: Basic concepts and clinical implications. Nature Reviews. Immunology. 2013;**13**(10):738-753

[52] Verma SK, Molitoris BA. Renal endothelial injury and microvascular dysfunction in acute kidney injury. Seminars in Nephrology. 2015;**35**(1):96-107

[53] Bouglé A, Duranteau J. Pathophysiology of sepsis-induced acute kidney injury: The role of global renal blood flow and renal vascular resistance. In: Kellum JA, Ronco C, Vincent JL, editors. Contributions to Nephrology. Karger AG; 2011. pp. 89-97. Available from: https://www.karger.com/Article/FullText/329243

[54] Lauby-Secretan B, Scoccianti C, Loomis D, Grosse Y, Bianchini F, Straif K. Body fatness and cancer – Viewpoint of the IARC working group. The New England Journal of Medicine. 2016;**375**(8):794-798

[55] Frisch CM, Zimmermann K, Zilleßen P, Pfeifer A, Racké K, Mayer P. Non-small cell lung cancer cell survival crucially depends on functional insulin receptors. Endocrine-Related Cancer. 2015;**22**(4):609-621

[56] Słabuszewska-Jóźwiak A, Lukaszuk A, Janicka-Kośnik M, Wdowiak A, Jakiel G. Role of leptin and adiponectin in endometrial Cancer. IJMS. 2022;**23**(10):5307

[57] Miethe C, Zamora M, Torres L, Raign KG, Groll CJ, Price RS. Characterizing the differential physiological effects of adipocytokines visfatin and resistin in liver cancer cells. Hormone Molecular Biology and Clinical Investigation. 2019;**2019**(2):38. DOI: 10.1515/hmbci-2018-0068/html

[58] Cunarro J, Casado S, Lugilde J, Tovar S. Hypothalamic mitochondrial dysfunction as a target in obesity and metabolic disease. Frontiers in Endocrinology. 2018;**9**:283

[59] Assumpção JAF, Pasquarelli-do-Nascimento G, Duarte MSV, Bonamino MH, Magalhães KG. The ambiguous role of obesity in oncology by promoting cancer but boosting antitumor immunotherapy. Journal of Biomedical Science. 2022;**29**(1):12

[60] Hauck AK, Huang Y, Hertzel AV, Bernlohr DA. Adipose oxidative stress and protein carbonylation. Journal of Biological Chemistry. 2019;**294**(4):1083-1088

[61] Jackisch L, Murphy AM, Kumar S, Randeva H, Tripathi G, McTernan PG. Tunicamycin-induced endoplasmic reticulum stress mediates mitochondrial dysfunction in human adipocytes. The Journal of Clinical Endocrinology & Metabolism. 2020;**105**(9):2905-2918

[62] Nishikawa M, Hashida M, Takakura Y. Catalase delivery for inhibiting ROS-mediated tissue injury and tumor metastasis. Advanced Drug Delivery Reviews. 2009;**61**(4):319-326

[63] Mondal S, Adhikari N, Banerjee S, Amin SA, Jha T. Matrix

metalloproteinase-9 (MMP-9) and its inhibitors in cancer: A minireview. European Journal of Medicinal Chemistry. 2020;**194**:112260

[64] Usman M, Volpi EV. DNA damage in obesity: Initiator, promoter and predictor of cancer. Mutation Research/Reviews in Mutation Research. 2018;**778**:23-37

[65] Quail DF, Dannenberg AJ. The obese adipose tissue microenvironment in cancer development and progression. Nature Reviews. Endocrinology. 2019;**15**(3):139-154

[66] Lu Y, Zhou XY, Zhou CL, Liu J, Yong T, Fan Y, et al. Insulin receptor tyrosine kinase substrate (IRTKS) promotes the tumorigenesis of pancreatic cancer via PI3K/AKT signaling. Human Cell. 2022;**35**(6):1885-1899

[67] Hu DX, Sun QF, Xu L, Lu HD, Zhang F, Li ZM, et al. Knockdown of DEAD-box 51 inhibits tumor growth of esophageal squamous cell carcinoma *via* the PI3K/AKT pathway. WJG. 2022;**28**(4):464-478

[68] Gu JW, Young E, Patterson SG, Makey KL, Wells J, Huang M, et al. Postmenopausal obesity promotes tumor angiogenesis and breast cancer progression in mice. Cancer Biology & Therapy. 2011;**11**(10):910-917

[69] Seo BR, Bhardwaj P, Choi S, Gonzalez J, Andresen Eguiluz RC, Wang K, et al. Obesity-dependent changes in interstitial ECM mechanics promote breast tumorigenesis. Science Translational Medicine. 2015;**2015**(7):301. DOI: 10.1126/scitranslmed.3010467

[70] Gonzalez-Perez R, Lanier V, Newman G. Leptin's pro-Angiogenic signature in breast cancer. Cancers. 2013;**5**(4):1140-1162

[71] Miethe C, Torres L, Zamora M, Price RS. Inhibition of PI3K/Akt and ERK signaling decreases visfatin-induced invasion in liver cancer cells. Hormone Molecular Biology and Clinical Investigation. 2021;**42**(4):357-366

[72] Ramos-Andrade I, Moraes J, Brandão-Costa RM, Vargas Da Silva S, De Souza A, Da Silva C, et al. Obese adipose tissue extracellular vesicles raise breast cancer cell malignancy. Endocrine-Related Cancer. 2020;**27**(10):571-582

[73] Dibaba DT, Judd SE, Gilchrist SC, Cushman M, Pisu M, Safford M, et al. Association between obesity and biomarkers of inflammation and metabolism with cancer mortality in a prospective cohort study. Metabolism. 2019;**94**:69-76

[74] Lathigara D, Kaushal D, Wilson RB. Molecular mechanisms of Western diet-induced obesity and obesity-related carcinogenesis—A narrative review. Metabolites. 2023;**13**(5):675

[75] Nigam M, Mishra AP, Deb VK, Dimri DB, Tiwari V, Bungau SG, et al. Evaluation of the association of chronic inflammation and cancer: Insights and implications. Biomedicine & Pharmacotherapy. 2023;**164**:115015

[76] Savic Vujovic K, Zivkovic A, Dozic I, Cirkovic A, Medic B, Srebro D, et al. Oxidative stress and inflammation biomarkers in postoperative pain modulation in surgically treated patients with laryngeal Cancer—Pilot study. Cell. 2023;**12**(10):1391

[77] Singh A, Mayengbam SS, Yaduvanshi H, Wani MR, Bhat MK. Obesity programs macrophages to support cancer progression. Cancer Research. 2022;**82**(23):4303-4312

[78] Oleinika K, Slisere B, Catalán D, Rosser EC. B cell contribution to

immunometabolic dysfunction and impaired immune responses in obesity. Clinical and Experimental Immunology. 2022;**210**(3):263-272

[79] Sharebiani H, Keramat S, Chavoshan A, Fazeli B, Stanek A. The influence of antioxidants on oxidative stress-induced vascular aging in obesity. Antioxidants. 2023;**12**(6):1295

[80] Luft VC, Schmidt MI, Pankow JS, Couper D, Ballantyne CM, Young JH, et al. Chronic inflammation role in the obesity-diabetes association: A case-cohort study. Diabetology and Metabolic Syndrome. 2013;**5**(1):31

[81] Russo S, Kwiatkowski M, Govorukhina N, Bischoff R, Melgert BN. Meta-inflammation and metabolic reprogramming of macrophages in diabetes and obesity: The importance of metabolites. Frontiers in Immunology. 2021;**12**:746151

[82] Wang G, Shen G, Jiang X, Chen Z, Yin T. Assessment of para-inflammation in a wound healing model. Experimental Therapy Medicine. 2020;**2020**:15. Available from: http://www.spandidos-publications.com/10.3892/etm.2020.8666

[83] Guarner V, Rubio-Ruiz ME. Low-grade systemic inflammation connects aging, metabolic syndrome and cardiovascular disease. In: Yashin AI, Jazwinski SM, editors. Interdisciplinary Topics in Gerontology and Geriatrics. S. Karger AG; 2015. pp. 99-106. Available from: https://www.karger.com/Article/FullText/364934

[84] Fülöp T, Larbi A, Witkowski JM. Human Inflammaging. Gerontology. 2019;**65**(5):495-504

[85] Lan T, Chen L, Wei X. Inflammatory cytokines in cancer: Comprehensive understanding and clinical Progress in gene therapy. Cell. 2021;**10**(1):100

[86] Upthegrove R, Khandaker GM. Cytokines, oxidative stress and cellular markers of inflammation in schizophrenia. In: Khandaker GM, Meyer U, Jones PB, editors. Neuroinflammation and Schizophrenia. Cham: Springer International Publishing; 2019. pp. 49-66. DOI: 10.1007/7854_2018_88

[87] Gusev E, Zhuravleva Y. Inflammation: A new look at an old problem. IJMS. 2022;**23**(9):4596

[88] Gusev EY, Zotova NV. Cellular stress and general pathological processes. CPD. 2019;**25**(3):251-297

[89] Gusev EY, Zhuravleva YA, Zotova NV. Correlation of the evolution of immunity and inflammation in vertebrates. Biology Bulletin Reviews. 2019;**9**(4):358-372

[90] Rather LJ. Disturbance of function (functio laesa): The legendary fifth cardinal sign of inflammation, added by Galen to the four cardinal signs of Celsus. Bulletin of the New York Academy of Medicine. 1971;**47**(3):303-322

[91] Tylutka A, Morawin B, Walas Ł, Michałek M, Gwara A, Zembron-Lacny A. Assessment of metabolic syndrome predictors in relation to inflammation and visceral fat tissue in older adults. Scientific Reports. 2023;**13**(1):89

[92] Antuña E, Cachán-Vega C, Bermejo-Millo JC, Potes Y, Caballero B, Vega-Naredo I, et al. Inflammaging: Implications in sarcopenia. IJMS. 2022;**23**(23):15039

[93] Martínez-Colón GJ, Ratnasiri K, Chen H, Jiang S, Zanley E, Rustagi A, et al. SARS-CoV-2 infection drives an inflammatory response in human adipose tissue through infection of adipocytes and macrophages. Science Translational Medicine. 2022;**14**(674):eabm9151

Chapter 6

Clinical Features of Multisystem Inflammatory Syndrome

Víctor Manuel Gutiérrez-Gómez, Beatriz Archundia-Jiménez, Rodrigo Miguel González-Sánchez, Jerónimo Amado López-Arriaga, Beatriz X. Pasco-Velázquez and Alejandra Gómez-Flores

Abstract

Multisystem inflammatory syndrome was first detected in pediatric patients in April 2020, related to COVID-19. The clinical manifestations are very broad and overlap with Kawasaki disease. Various organizations have developed guides with case definitions in order to facilitate diagnosis and epidemiological reporting. In this chapter, we present the clinical manifestations of multisystem inflammatory syndrome, considering the case definition of various organizations and case series reports, systematic reviews, and meta-analyses. We also address multisystem inflammatory syndrome in adults in the neonatal period.

Keywords: MIS-C, MIS-A, multisystemic inflammatory syndrome, MIS-N, PIMS-TS

1. Introduction

Multisystem inflammatory syndrome (MIS) is a set of symptoms caused by an extreme inflammatory response related to coronavirus disease 2019 (COVID-19) and was first detected in Europe between April and May 2020. The Royal College of Pediatrics and Child Health (RCPCH) of the United Kingdom (UK) referred to this acute condition as pediatric inflammatory multisystem temporally associated with COVID-19 (PIMS-TS). A few days later, the World Health Organization (WHO) and the Center for Disease Control and Prevention (CDC) named it multisystem inflammatory syndrome in children (MIS-C). In June 2020, multisystem inflammatory syndrome was also reported in adults (MIS-A). In June 2021, neonatal multisystem inflammatory syndrome was described (MIS-N) [1–3].

2. Multisystem inflammatory syndrome in children (MIS-C)

The first cases of COVID-19 due to SARS-CoV-2 in children manifested as mild illness. In April 2020, cases of some children with positive SARS-CoV-2 who presented a severe hyperinflammatory state were reported, considered to be Kawasaki disease (KD), sepsis, bacterial syndromes, or toxic shock, among other diagnoses. This syndrome was called MISC-C, and due to difficulty in establishing the diagnosis, various organizations such as RCPCH, WHO, and CDC, with the opinion of experts, developed documents with the aim of identifying cases and providing advice to doctors on the management of these patients. All of these documents present a case definition that includes clinical manifestations (**Table 1**).

Dufort et al. [6] reported a case series of 99 patients with MIS-C, younger than 21 years old, admitted to New York hospitals from March 1 through May 10, 2020. Of the 99 patients, 54% were male, 31% of the patients were 0 to 5 years of age, 42% were between 6 and 12 years of age, and 26% were between 13 and 20 years of age. Regarding race, it was found that of 78 patients, 37% were white, 40% were black, and 23% were of other races. Regarding the ethnic group of 85 patients, 36% were Hispanic. Of the 36 patients who presented comorbidities, 29 of them were obese. The 99 patients presented the following symptoms upon admission: fever or chills 100%, chest pain 11%, abdominal pain 61%, nausea or vomiting 58%, diarrhea 49%, rash 60%, swollen hands or feet 9%, conjunctivitis 56%, mucosal changes 27%, headache 29%, altered mental status or confusion 2%, lymphadenopathy 6%, muscle aches or myalgias 17%, joint pain 4%, congestion 13%, sore throat 16%, cough 31%, shortness of breath 19%, wheezing 1%. The vital sign values were; median heart rate 133 beats/min (range: 120–148 beats/min), tachycardia 97%, median respiratory rate 27 breaths/min (range: 23–36 breaths/min), tachypnea 78%, hypotension 32%, median temperature 38.3°C (range: 37.5–39.3°C), temperature ≥ 38.0°C 63%, median oxygen saturation 98 (range: 97–100)%, oxygen saturation < 92% 4% [6].

Davies et al. [7] conducted a multicenter observational study of pediatric patients hospitalized in PICU in the United Kingdom between April 1 and May 10, 2020, who met the requirements of the PIMS-TS case definition published by the RCPCH. Seventy-eight cases of PIMS-TS were reported by 21 of 23 PICUs. Of the 78 patients, 67% were male, with a median age of 11 years (range: 8–14 years). The clinical presenting features were: fever 100%, shock 87% (vasodilated 71%, vasoconstricted 17%), abdominal pain 62%, diarrhea 64%, vomiting 63%, any abdominal symptom (pain, diarrhea, or vomiting) 90%, rash 45%, conjunctivitis 29% [7].

In a systematic literature review that included 56 studies, Yousef et al found 646 pediatric patients diagnosed with MIS-C between April 2020 and October 2020. The average age was 10 years (between 0.5–17 years); 52.2% were male. Of the 646, 51.1% of the cases occurred in the United States, 21.4% were presented in the UK, 8.7% were presented in France and Switzerland combined, and 18.9% were presented in other countries. Of the total patients, 99.5% presented fever, recording an average "max temperature" of 39.4°C (between 38.2 and 41°C). The average duration of fever before presentation to hospital was 5 days (range: 1–12 days).

The frequency of other symptoms was: generalized abdominal pain 77.6%, vomiting 75.4%, diarrhea 63.2%, dyspnea 80%, coryza 60%, cough 55%, sora throat 17%, chest pain 13.6%, headache 30.4%, irritability 57.4%, fatigue 61.5%, and myalgia 16.8%. On physical examination: hypotension 49.7%, tachycardia 93.5%, 67.3% tachypnea, polymorphic rash 57.6%, non-exudative bilateral conjunctivitis 52.9%, lip/oral cavity cracking 37%, hand and feet anomalies 26%, pharyngeal erythema, unilateral cervical lymphadenopathy 13.1%. Abdominal tenderness 51.9%, meningeal signs 21.2%, and bilateral crackles on auscultation 15% [8].

In a system review and meta-analysis, Santos et al. selected 98 studies (2275 patients with MIS-C) published between December 1, 2019, and July 10, 2021.

	RCPCH [1]	WHO [2]	CDC [3]	CSTE/CDC [4]	Molloy et al. [5]
Publication date	May 1, 2020	May, 2020	May, 2020	January, 2023	May, 2023
Denomination	PIMS-TS	MIS-C	MIS-C	MIS-C	MIS-C
Patient age (years)	Child	0–19	<21	<21	<21
Abdominal pain	S	S			S
Cardiac hypotension	M	S			S
Cardiac manifestations			S		S
Confusion	S				S
Conjunctivitis	S	S		S	S
Coronary abnormalities		S			S
Cough	S				S
Dermal manifestations			S		S
Diarrhea	S	S			S
Erythema of the hands or feet				S	S
Fever	A >38.5° C Persistent	A ≥ 3 days	A ≥38.0°C for 24 hours, Subjective lasting ≥24 hours.	A ≥38.0° C documented or subjective.	A ≥38.0° C for ≥ days. Subjective lasting ≥3 days.
Gastrointestinal manifestations			S		S
Headache	S				S
Hematologic manifestations			S		S
Inflammation of the oral mucosa				S	S
Kidney manifestations			S		S
Lymphadenopathy	S				S
Mucus membrane changes	S	S			S
Myocardial dysfunction		S			S
Neck swelling	S				
Neurological manifestations			S		S
Oxygen requirement	M				

	RCPCH [1]	WHO [2]	CDC [3]	CSTE/CDC [4]	Molloy et al. [5]
Pericardial effusion					S
Pericarditis					S
Rash	S	S		S	S
Resp symptoms	S	S			S
Seizures					S
Shock		S			S
Sore throat	S				S
Swollen hands and feet	S	S		S	S
Syncope	S				
Valvulitis (cardiac)		S			S
Vomiting	S	S			
Without another diagnosis that justifies the clinical manifestations and laboratory and imaging findings.	A	A	A	A	A
COVID-19 evidence.	The polymerase chain reaction (PCR) test positive or negative	Evidence or likely contact	Evidence or likely contact (4 weeks prior)	Detection or close contact (up to 2 months prior)	Evidence or recent exposure
No alternative plausible diagnoses					

A: all—present in all patients; M: most—present in most patients; S: some—present in some of patients.

Table 1.
Clinical manifestations of MIS-C included in case definition of various organizations.

The median age was 8.9 years (range: 0.1 days to 20 years old), and 58% were male. The symptom and clinical characteristics were: fever 100%, gastrointestinal symptoms (not specifics) 82%, abdominal pain 68%, vomiting 66%, cardiac symptoms 66%, shock 60%, hypotension 59%, erythema 59%, diarrhea 58%, conjunctivitis 54%, cough 41%, respiratory symptoms 39%, comorbidity 33%, dyspnea 29%, headache 28%, neurologic symptoms 28%, and sore throat 20% [9].

Jiang et al. did a live systematic review including a schedule of activities covering the period from December 1, 2019, to July 31, 2021. A total of 123 studies that met all the requirements for the final descriptive and risk factor analyses were included, with a total population size of 4475 children with MIS-C. The mean age of MIS-C patients was 8.1 ± 2.37 years, and 58.11% (1856/3184, 95% CI 56.40–59.82%) were boys. Among the 2841 individuals with race/ethnicity data, African black was 24.89%, Hispanic white 25.18%, Asian 23.41%, and non-Hispanic white 19.01%. Prevalent clinical symptoms observed in MIS-C cases were fever 90.85%, not-specified gastrointestinal symptoms 51.98%, rash 49..63%, abdominal pain 48.97%, conjunctivitis 46.93%, vomiting 43.79%, respiratory symptoms 41.75%, diarrhea 40.10%, pharyngeal erythema 31.91%, myocarditis 29.34%, neurologic symptoms 26.92%, erythema and edema of hands and feet 21.00%, and cervical lymphadenopathy 19.11%. Diagnostic criteria of incomplete KD 18.67%, complete KD 15.18%. Shock 37.75% [10].

Table 2 shows the frequency of signs and symptoms of MIS-C presented by the groups of patients reported by previously mentioned authors.

3. Multisystem inflammatory syndrome in adults (MIS-A)

In June 2020, a multisystem inflammatory syndrome in adults (MIS-A) was mentioned for the first time, and subsequently, multiple cases have been reported. In MIS-A, it is considered that an abnormal immune repose occurs in a SARS-CoV-2 infection, with various symptoms, usually fever, systemic inflammation that can affect several organs and shock [11, 12].

3.1 CDC case definition for MIS-A

In 2021, through expert opinion, the CDC developed a case definition of MIS-A [11]. The clinical manifestations of this definition are presented in **Table 3**.

In a series of 16 cases in patients between 21 and 50 years of age, nine were woman. Seven had some underlying disease (6/16 obese, 2/12 diabetic, 2/16 hypertension, and 1/16 obstructive sleep apnea). Eight patients had documented respiratory illnesses before developing MIS-A symptoms, and eight did not. The initial symptoms and signs that this group of patients presented were fever (75%), cardiac symptoms such as chest pain or palpitations (37.5%), manifestations of cardiac disorders (100%), gastrointestinal symptoms (81.2%), dermatological manifestations (31.2%), including mucositis (18.7%) [12].

In a review of 36 documented cases of MIS-A, the mean age of patients was 33 years, with male predominance (63%). Contracted SARS-CoV-2 infection (47%), suggested by CRP, antibody testing, or clinically. Fever (86%). Gastrointestinal symptoms: nausea (19%), abdominal pain (30%), vomiting (13%), and diarrhea (19%). Sore throat (14%), unilateral cervical pain/swelling (16$). Some patients had predominant visual symptoms. Tachycardia (61%) and hypotension/cardiogenic shock with documented impaired ejection fraction (64%) [13].

4. Multisystem inflammatory syndrome in neonates

Pawar et al. introduced the MIS-N and neonatal MIS-C labels. The MIS-N label was created to differentiate newborns who present with multisystem inflammatory syndrome in the first week after birth secondary to possible maternal COVID-19 infection, with passive transmission of antibodies. Neonatal MIS-C is used to identify newborns who had neonatal, early-onset, or late-onset COVID-19 and who subsequently, between the second and fourth weeks after birth, developed multisystem inflammation. Both MIS-N and neonatal MIS-C are relatively rare [14].

Their case series included 20 suspected MIS-N neonates born to mothers with a history of SARS-CoV-2 infection or exposure to COVID-19 patients. They admitted to seven NICUs in Kolhapur between September 1, 2020, and April 30, 2023. The median maternal age was 26.5 years (range 20–34 years). 20% of the patients were premature <33 weeks, 65% were between 34 and 36 weeks, and

Clinical manifestation	Dufort et al. [6] (99 cases)	Davies et al. [7] (78 cases)	Yousef et al. [8] (56 studies, 646 cases)	Santos et al. [9] (98 studies, 2275 cases)	Jiang et al. [10] (123 studies, 4475 cases)
Fever	100%	100%	99.5%	100%	90.85%
Gastrointestinal symptoms	—	90%	—	82%	51.98%
Abdominal tenderness	—	—	51.9%	—	—
Abdominal paint	61%	62%	77.6%	68%	48.97%
Nausea	58%	—	—	—	—
Vomiting		63%	75.4%	66%	43.79%
Diarrhea	49%	64%	63.2%	58%	40.1%
Rash	60%	45%	57.6%	59%	49.63%
Erythema and edema of hands or feet	9%	—	26%	—	21%
Conjunctivitis	56%	29%	52.9%	54%	46.93%
Coryza	—	—	60%	—	—
Mucosal changes	27%	—	—	—	—
Lip/oral cavity cracking	—	—	37%	—	—
Neurologic symptoms	—	—	—	28%	26.92%
Headache	29%	—	30.4%	28%	—
Confusion	2%	—	—	—	—
Irritability	—	—	57.4%	—	—
Meningeal signs	—	—	21.2%	—	—
Cervical lymphadenopathy	6%	—	13%	—	19.11%
Myalgias	17%	—	16.8%	—	—
Joint pain	4%	—	—	—	—
Fatigue	—	—	61.5%	—	—
Respiratory symptoms	—	—	—	39%	41.75%
Congestion	13%	—	—	—	—
Sore throat	16%	—	17%	20%	—
Pharyngeal erythema	—	—	13%	—	31.91%
Cough	31%	—	55%	41%	—
Shortness of breath	19%	—	—	—	—
Dyspnea	—	—	80%	29%	—
Wheezing	1%	—	—	—	—
Chest paint	11%	—	13.6%	—	—
Bilateral crackles on auscultation	—	—	15%	—	—
Tachypnea	79%	—	—	—	—
Oxygen saturation < 92%	4%	—	—	—	—

Clinical manifestation	Dufort et al. [6] (99 cases)	Davies et al. [7] (78 cases)	Yousef et al. [8] (56 studies, 646 cases)	Santos et al. [9] (98 studies, 2275 cases)	Jiang et al. [10] (123 studies, 4475 cases)
Tachycardia	97%	—	93.5%	—	
Cardiac symptoms	—	—	—	66%	—
Hypotension	32%	—	49.7%	59%	—
Shock	—	87%	—	60%	37.75%

Table 2.
Frequency of signs and symptoms of MIS-C in groups of patients reported by various authors [6–10].

15% were term. There was no difference in distribution by sex. The most frequent clinical manifestations were heart disease, present in 18 (90%) patients (once they had rhythm disorders). Only two newborns (10%) presented fever (both on the first day of life). Eleven patients (55%) had respiratory manifestations. Eight newborns required mechanical ventilation, and three required CPAP. Six (30%) patients had gastrointestinal manifestations. Feeding intolerance and gastric aspirates were seen in six neonates. Two had lower gastrointestinal bleeding. A newborn died [14].

In a systematic review that included 13 papers, 33 cases of newborns with MIS-N were described; 72.7% were premature between 33 and 36 weeks (mean 34 weeks). The average birth weight was 2020 (1890–2620) grams. In all patients, the diagnosis was made in the first 3 days of life, with an average stay of 16 days. The clinical manifestations were fever at 18.2%, cardiovascular at 78.8%, respiratory difficulty at 66.7%, gastrointestinal at 27.3%, neurological at 24.2%, and acute kidney injury at 15.2%. The outcome was favorable in 30 neonates (90.9%). Two neonates die, one from multiple organ dysfunction and the other from necrotizing enterocolitis [15].

Based on the classification of clinical manifestations of COVID-19 in the neonatal period developed by Lakshminrusimha et al. [16], Molloy et al. [5] recommend using the terms early neonatal COVID-19, Late neonatal COVID-19, MIS-N, and MIS-C:

- Early neonatal COVID-19: neonate <7 days after birth at disease manifestation, with respiratory distress, apnea, or asymptomatic, with positive RT-PCR or antigen test from neonate after first few hours (source of SARS-CoV-2 infection: mother).

- Late neonatal COVID-19: age of neonate at disease manifestation typically, 2–3 weeks after birth, with respiratory distress, congestion, apnea, fever. With positive RT-PCR or antigen test from neonate (source of SARS-CoV-2 infection: family members including mother).

- MIS-N: neonate <7 days after birth at disease manifestation, with a neonatal inflammatory illness involving ≥2 organ system involvement (cardiac, gastrointestinal, hematologic, renal, respiratory, and neurological clinic manifestations), suggesting not include fever (which is relatively uncommon in neonates), along with the maternal history of SARS-CoV-2 infection during pregnancy (source of SARS-CoV-2 infection: mother).

Age	> 21 years
Hospitalization	> 24 hours
Fever	> 38.0°C or subjective. > 24 hours before or in the initial 3 days of hospitalization.
At least three criteria (one of them primary)	
Primary criteria	Cardiac (serious illness): • Myocarditis. • Pericarditis. • Coronary dilation/aneurysm. • Ventricular dysfunction (left or right). • Second or third-degree atrioventricular block. • Ventricular tachycardia.
	Rash, Non-purulent conjunctivitis.
Secondary criteria	Neurological (new appearance): • Encephalopathy. • Seizures. • Meningeal signs. • Peripheral neuropathy.
	Hypotension or shock.
	Gastrointestinal: • Abdominal pain. • Vomiting. • Diarrhea.
	Thrombocytopenia (< 150,000/microliter).
No other diagnosis.	
Evidence of SARS-CoV-2 infection (current or recent).	

Table 3.
MIS-A case definition developed by the CDC [11].

- MIS-C: age of neonate at disease manifestation typically, 2–6 weeks after birth, with neonatal inflammatory illness involving ≥2 organ system involvement (cardiac, gastrointestinal, hematologic, renal, respiratory, and neurological clinic manifestations) and fever (source of SARS-CoV-2-infection: self, neonate with neonatal COVID with or without clinical signs).

5. Comparison with Kawasaki disease (KD)

The MIS-C diagnostic clinical features are general and overlap with those of KD. MIS-C has specific characteristics: it predominates in older children and most frequently affects the respiratory and digestive systems. Patients may present with abdominal pain, vomiting, diarrhea, shock, cardiac complication (myocarditis, left ventricular dysfunction, valvular regurgitation, pericardial effusion, and pericarditis) and have fewer symptoms of conjunctivitis. KD is an acute systemic vasculitis that predominantly affects children under 5 years of age and whose etiology is unknown [17–19].

Table 4 shows the similarities and differences between MIS-C and Kawasaki disease (KD).

Although the presence of a positive test for SARS-CoV-2 is more suggestive of MIS-C, it can also trigger KD in some patients. A positive SARS-CoV-2 antibody test is more difficult to interpret at this given widespread infection and vaccination [5].

Kostik et al. [18] created a score to discriminate MIS-C from KD, which includes five criteria:

- C-reactive protein >11 mg/dl—18 points
- D-dimer >607 ng/ml—27 points
- Patient >5 years—30 points
- Low platelets—25 points
- Gastrointestinal manifestations—28 points

A score > 55 points discriminates MIS-C from KD. This scale has a sensitivity of 87.5% and a specificity of 89.1% [19].

MIS-A shares many similarities with KD. To establish the diagnosis of KD, the patient must present fever for >5 days and at least four of the following signs:

- Conjunctivitis,
- Oropharyngeal mucositis or IgA infiltration of the upper respiratory tract,
- Cervical lymphadenopathy,
- Skin erythema,
- Edema or erythema of the extremities.

KD can present with acute kidney damage or the presence of aneurysms, especially in the abdominal aorta and coronary arteries [13].

To establish the diagnosis of COVID-19 Kawasaki-like syndrome, during or after COVID-19 infection and having ruled out other infections as a cause, the patient must have a fever for >3 days, and at least two of the following signs:

- Rash,
- Hypotension or shock,
- Acute cardiac injury.

Also present coagulation disorders, or acute gastrointestinal symptoms. With elevation of inflammatory markers (CRP, D-dimer, and/or ferritin) [13].

Similarities between MIS-C and KD	
Fever Mucous membrane changes Rash Conjunctivitis Lymphadenopathy Frequent cardiac involvement Laboratory tests demonstrating significant inflammation	
Differences between MIS-C and KD	
MIS-C	**KD**
• Age of affected patients: 5–13 years. • More likely to have gastrointestinal manifestations: abdominal pain, vomiting, and diarrhea. • Some patients have developed coronary artery dilatation aneurysms (complete resolution at follow-up). • Depressed ventricular function and highly elevated brain peptide (BNP) are more typical of MIS-C. • Normal blood cell count, lymphopenia, and thrombocytopenia. • Troponin increased. • Brain natriuretic peptide increased.	• Age of affected patients: <5 years. • Coronary artery aneurysms or dilation and pericardial effusion are most common. • White blood cell count, lymphocytosis, neutrophilia, and thrombocytosis. • Troponin usually normal. • Brain natriuretic peptide usually normal.

Table 4.
MIS-C and KC: Similarities and differences [5, 17].

6. Conclusion

Multisystem inflammatory syndrome is a rare disease with a large number of clinical manifestations, both in pediatric, adult, and neonatal presentations. The studies carried out have allowed us to identify the weight of each sign and symptom for the establishment of a timely diagnosis. Without a doubt, clinical guidelines and case definitions will be adjusted as research on this entity continues.

Acknowledgements

We thank Dr. Nicolas Padilla Raygoza for allowing us to participate in this book and Laura Divic for the support provided during the editorial process.

Conflict of interest

The authors declare no conflict of interest.

Nomenclature

CDC	Center for Disease Control and Prevention
CPAP	continuous positive airway pressure
CRP	C-reactive protein

CSTE/CDC	Council of State and Territorial Epidemiologists/CDC
KD	Kawasaki disease
MIS-A	multisystem inflammatory syndrome in adults
MIS-C	multisystem inflammatory syndrome in children
MIS-N	neonatal multisystem inflammatory syndrome
NICU	Neonatal Intensive Care Unit
PICU	Pediatric Intensive Care Unit
PIMS-TS	pediatric inflammatory multisystem temporally associated with COVID-19
RCPCH	Royal College of Pediatrics and Child Health
RT-PCR	reverse transcription polymerase chain reaction
WHO	World Health Organization

Author details

Víctor Manuel Gutiérrez-Gómez[1,2*], Beatriz Archundia-Jiménez[3], Rodrigo Miguel González-Sánchez[4], Jerónimo Amado López-Arriaga[1], Beatriz X. Pasco-Velázquez[1,2] and Alejandra Gómez-Flores[1,2]

1 School of Medicine, Autonomous Mexico State University, Toluca, Mexico

2 Maternal and Child Institute of the State of Mexico, Toluca, Mexico

3 Regional General Hospital 220, Mexican Social Security Institute, Toluca, Mexico

4 School of Medicine, Autonomous University of Queretaro, Queretaro, Mexico

*Address all correspondence to: victor.gutierrezg@hotmail.com

References

[1] Royal College of Paediatric and Child Health. Guidance: Pediatric Multisystem Inflammatory Syndrome Temporally Associated with COVID-19. 2020. Available from: https://www.rcpch.ac.uk/sites/default/files/2020-05/COVID-19-Paediactric-multisystem-%20inflammatory%20syndrome-20200501.pdf

[2] World Health Organization. Multisystem inflammatory syndrome in children and adolescents temporally related to COVID-19. Scientific Brief. 15 May 2020. WHO reference number: WHO/2019-nCoV/Sci_Brief/Multisystem_Syndrome_Children/2020.1. Available from: //iris.who.int/bitstream/handle/10665/332095/WHO-2019-nCoV-Sci_Brief-Multisystem_Syndrome_Children-2020.1-eng.pdf?sequence=1

[3] Centers for Disease Control and Prevention. Multisystem Inflammatory Syndrome in Children (MIS-C) Associated with Coronavirus Disease 2019 (COVID-19). 2020. Available from: https://emergency.cdc.gov/han/2020/han00432.asp

[4] Melgar M, Lee EH, Miller AD, Lim S, Brown CM, Yousaf AR, et al. Council of State and Territorial Epidemiologists/CDC surveillance case definition for multisystem inflammatory syndrome in children associated with SARS-CoV-2 infection – United States. MMWR. 2022;**71**(4):1-14

[5] Molloy EJ, Nakra N, Gale C, Dimitriades VR, Lakshminrusimha S. Multisystem inflammatory syndrome in children (MIS-C) and neonates (MIS-N) associated with COVID-19: Optimizing definition and management. Pediatric Research. 2023;**93**(6):1499-1508. DOI: 10.1038/s41390-022-02263-w

[6] Dufort EM, Koumans EH, Chow EJ, Rosenthal EM, Muse A, Rowlands J, et al. Multisystem inflammatory syndrome in children in New York state. The New England Journal of Medicine. 2020;**383**:347-358. DOI: 10.1056/NEJMoa2021756

[7] Davies P, Evans C, Kanthimathinathan HK, Lillie J, Brierly J, Waters G, et al. Intensive care admission of children temporally associated with SARS-CoV-2 (PIMS-TS) in the UK: A multicentre observational study. Lancet Child and Adolescent Health. 2020;**4**:669-677. DOI: 10.1016/S2352-4642(20)30215-7

[8] Yousef MS, Idris NA, Yap C, Alsubaie AA, Kakodkar P. Systematic review on the clinical presentation and management of the COVID-19 associated multisystem inflammatory syndrome in children (MIS-C). AIMS Allergy and Immunology. 2021;**5**(1):38-55. DOI: 10.3932/Allergy.2021004

[9] Santos MO, Goncalves LC, Silva PA, Moreira AL, ITO CR, Peixoto FA. Multisystem inflammatory syndrome (MIS-C): A systematic review and meta-analysis of clinical characteristics, treatment, and outcomes. Journal de Pediatria. 2022;**98**(4):338-349. DOI: 10.1016/j.jped.2021.08.006

[10] Li J, Tang K, Infan O, Li X, Zhang E, Bhutta Z. Epidemiology, clinical features, and outcomes of multisystem inflammatory syndrome in children (MIS-C) and adolescents – A live systematic review and meta-analysis. Current Pediatric Report. 2022;**10**:19-30. DOI: 10.1007/s40124-022-00264-1

[11] Centers for Disease Control and Prevention. Multisystem Inflammatory

Syndrome in Adults (MIS-A) Case Definition and Information for Healthcare Providers. Available from: https://www.cdc.gov/mis/mis-a/hcp.html

[12] Morris SB, Schwartz NG, Patel P, Abbo L, Beauchamps L, Balan S, et al. Case series of multisystem inflammatory syndrome in adults associated with SARS-CoV-2 infection – United Kingdom and United States, March–August 2020. MMWR. 2020;**69**(40):1450-1456

[13] Behzadi F, Ulloa NA, Danckers M. Multisystem inflammatory syndrome in adults: A case report and review of the literature. Journal of Medical Case Report. 2022;**16**:102-121. DOI: 10.1186/s13256-022-03295-w

[14] Pawar R, Gavade V, Patil N, Mali V, Girwalkar A, Tarkasband V, et al. Neonatal multisystem inflammatory syndrome (MIS-N) associated with prenatal maternal SARS-CoV-2: A case series. The Child. 2021;**8**:572. DOI: 10.3390/children8070572

[15] De Rose DU, Pugnaloni F, Cali M, Ronci S, Caoci S, Maddaloni C, et al. Multisystem inflammatory syndrome in neonates born to mothers with SARC-CoV-2 infection (MIS-N) and in neonates and infants younger than 6 months with acquired COVID-19 (MIS-C): A systematic review. Viruses. 2022;**14**:750. DOI: 10.3390/v14040750

[16] Lakshminrusimha S, Hudak ML, Dimitriades VR, Higgins RD. Multisystem inflammatory syndrome in neonates following maternal SARS-CoV-2 COVID-19 infection. American Journal of Perinatology. 2022;**39**:1166-1171. DOI: 10.1055/a-1682-3075

[17] Waseem M, Shariff MA, Ty ET, Mortel D, Savadkar S, Lee H, et al. Multisystem inflammatory syndrome in children. The Journal of Emergency Medicine. 2021;**62**(1):28-37. DOI: 10.1016/j.emermed.2021.07.070

[18] Kostik MM, Bregel LV, Avrusin IS, Dondurei EA, Matyunova AE, Efrenova OS, et al. Distinguishing between multisystem inflammatory syndrome, associated with COVID-19 in children and the Kawasaki disease; development of preliminary criteria based on the data of the retrospective multicenter cohort study. Front Pediatr. 10 Nov 2021;**9**:787353. DOI: 10.3380/fped.2021.787353

[19] Tong T, Yao X, Lin Z, Tao Y, Xu J, Xu X, et al. Similarities and differences between MIS-C and KD: A systematic review and meta-analysis. Pediatric Rheumatology. 2022;**20**:112. DOI: 10.1186/s12969-022-0771-x

Chapter 7

Clinical Data, Complications, Sequelae, and Death Causes in MIS-C

Alije Keka-Sylaj

Abstract

Multisystem inflammatory syndrome in children (MIS-C) is a potentially life-threatening childhood disease caused by severe acute respiratory syndrome coronavirus 2 (SARS-CoV-2) infection, manifested by the persistence of fever and multiple organ dysfunction, elevated inflammatory markers, and the lack of an alternative diagnosis. Generally, at the time of diagnosis, children had positive antibodies to SARS-CoV-2 but negative nasopharyngeal SARS-CoV-2 polymerase chain reaction (PCR) tests at the time of the MIS-C evaluation. Fever, gastrointestinal, cardiovascular, hematologic, mucocutaneous, and respiratory manifestations are common clinical features. Patients with MIS-C are typically previously healthy, and their most common comorbidity is obesity. Cardiovascular abnormalities, which are the most prevalent complications of MIS-C patients, and thromboembolic events have the greatest influence on the severity of the disease. The majority of patients with MIS-C have a severe course of the disease, requiring intensive care unit admission up to 76%, respiratory support, special care, and vigorous treatment including inotropic drugs; nonetheless, the majority of patients have favorable outcomes, and overall mortality is low.

Keywords: manifestations, complications, comorbidities, sequelae, death, MIS-C

1. Introduction

Multisystem inflammatory syndrome in children (MIS-C) began to be reported in April 2020 as a new and potentially life-threatening childhood disease that has been temporarily associated with the severe acute respiratory syndrome coronavirus 2 (SARS-CoV-2) [1].

This condition commonly manifests 2–6 weeks after a typically mild or asymptomatic infection with SARS-CoV-2, with a variety of clinical presentations, the majority of which include persistent fever, multisystem organ involvement, and elevated inflammatory markers in the absence of an alternative diagnosis [2].

Following the publication of these unusual patient presentations, the Centers for Disease Control and Prevention (CDC) and the World Health Organization (WHO) in May 2020 provided a case definition of this disorder based on clinical manifestations, laboratory features, and findings from additional exams. This disorder was named multisystem inflammatory syndrome in children (MIS-C) associated with COVID-19 2023 [3, 4].

The case definition was updated by the Council of State and Territorial Epidemiologists (CSTE) and the Centers for Disease Control and Prevention (CDC) by developing a new MIS-C surveillance case definition, corresponding case report form, and case report form guidance document to be used starting January 1, 2023 [3].

This case definition includes any illness in a person aged less than 21 years who meets

- the clinical and the laboratory criteria (confirmed), or
- the clinical criteria and epidemiologic linkage criteria (probable), or
- the vital records criteria (suspect)

The clinical criteria in this case definition include.

An illness characterized by all of the following, in the absence of a more likely alternative diagnosis.

- subjective or documented fever (temperature $\geq$ 38.0°C)
- clinical severity requiring hospitalization or resulting in death
- evidence of systemic inflammation indicated by C-reactive protein $\geq$3.0 mg/dL (30 mg/L)

New onset manifestations in at least two of the following categories:

Cardiac involvement indicated by

- left ventricular ejection fraction <55% or
- coronary artery dilatation, aneurysm, or ectasia, or
- troponin elevated above laboratory normal range or indicated as elevated in a clinical note

Mucocutaneous involvement indicated by

- rash or
- inflammation of the oral mucosa (e.g., mucosal erythema or swelling, drying or fissuring of the lips, strawberry tongue), or
- conjunctivitis or conjunctival injection (redness of the eyes), or
- extremity findings (e.g., erythema [redness] or edema [swelling] of the hands or feet)
- shock

DOI: http://dx.doi.org/10.5772/intechopen.1003727

Gastrointestinal involvement indicated by

- abdominal pain, or
- vomiting, or
- diarrhea

Hematologic involvement indicated by

- platelet count <150,000 cells/μL, or
- absolute lymphocyte count (ALC) < 1000 cells/μL.

The clinical criteria of case definition of MIS-C according to the World Health Organization [4] include children and adolescents 0–19 years of age with fever >3 days and two of the following:

- rash or bilateral non-purulent conjunctivitis or muco-cutaneous inflammation signs (oral, hands or feet)
- hypotension or shock
- features of myocardial dysfunction, pericarditis, valvulitis, or coronary abnormalities (including ECHO findings or elevated Troponin/NT-proBNP)
- evidence of coagulopathy (by prothrombin time-PT , partial thromboplastin time- PTT , elevated d-Dimers)
- acute gastrointestinal problems (diarrhea, vomiting, or abdominal pain)

2. Clinical features of multisystem inflammatory syndrome in children

MIS-C symptoms generally appear 2–6 weeks after infection, and it is common that children with MIS-C would have had no or a few symptoms of COVID-19 [5]. MIS-C seems to develop in the post-infectious stage rather than during the acute infection stage of COVID-19 [6].

With the rapid spread of the COVID-19 pandemic, a considerable number of MIS-C cases have been reported from almost every country in the world with varying clinical manifestations. A large number of MIS-C-related publications include systematic reviews and meta-analyses that present clinical data, complications, and outcomes of more than a hundred MIS-C cases [6–15].

According to these studies, males and children aged 7–9 years have a higher risk of developing MIS-C than other age groups and females overall, as shown in **Table 1**.

Most patients with MIS-C do not have any reported underlying medical condition, but in those who do, obesity is the most common [7–11].

The percentage of reported comorbidities in those studies varies from approximately 3–40% [10, 13]. Apart from obesity being the most frequent, other

Author	Studies included	Number of MIS-C cases	Median age (years)	Gender dominance
Jiang et al., [6]	123	4475	8.1	Male (58.11%)
Santos et al., [7]	48	2144	8.9	Male (58%)
Hoste et al., [8]	68	953	8.4	Male (58.9%)
Radia et al., [9]	35	783	8.6	Male (56%)
Ahmed et al., [10]	39	662	9.3	Male (52.3%)
Dhar et al., [11]	18	883	8.9	Male (56%)
Kornitzer et al., [12]	54	543	8.9	Male (56%)
Williams et al., [13]	18	833	9	Male (57%)
Sood et al., [14]	17	992	7	Male (57%)
Miller et al., [15]	Reported case	4470	9	Male (59.9%)

Table 1.
The characteristics of the study sample by gender and age group.

comorbidities reported include endocrine (diabetes, hypothyroidism, congenital adrenal hyperplasia), respiratory (asthma, chronic pulmonary disease), gastrointestinal (Crohn's disease), cardiovascular disease, neurologic/behavioral, liver or kidney disease, immunocompromised or immunodeficiency, cancer, immunologic/allergic, hematologic, coexisting infections, acute leukemia, glucose-6-phosphate dehydrogenase deficiency [7–11].

Patients with MIS-C usually present with persistent fever, abdominal pain, vomiting, diarrhea, skin rash, mucocutaneous lesions or KD-like symptoms and, in severe cases, with hypotension and shock or toxic shock syndrome [15, 16]. Some patients develop myocarditis, cardiac dysfunction, and acute kidney injury [6, 10, 13–15].

The most common symptoms in reported MIS-C cases [6–15] are as follows:

Persistent fever, sometimes lasting 3 or 4 days, as a key criterion in the definition of MIS-C, was reported in almost all cases, from 85 to 100%.

Gastrointestinal involvement or symptoms mimicking viral gastroenteritis or mesenteric lymphadenitis are very frequent in 46–86% of cases, including abdominal pain up to 74%, vomiting up to 68%, and diarrhea up to 53%, whereas loss of appetite, emesis, and poor oral intake are less frequent (7–18%).

Cardiovascular involvement or manifestations are frequently seen in patients with MIS-C (23–65%) and manifest as tachycardia (20–56%), myocarditis (13–65%), mild to moderate decreased left ventricular ejection fraction (22–61%), pericardial effusions (15–47%), and abnormalities, dilatation, or aneurysms of the coronary arteries (11–35%).

Most MIS-C patients present with hypotension; in addition, a larger proportion of MIS-C patients (21–65%) developed hemodynamic shock or toxic shock, which is the main reason for using inotropic support.

The majority of MIS-C cases (38–58%) show mucocutaneous involvement or KD-like features, including erythema or rash (20–58%), non-purulent conjunctivitis or conjunctival injection (25–52%), tongue swelling (5–31%), polymorphous exanthema (49%), erythema and edema or swollen of hands and feet (21%), and cheilitis (33%).

Patients with MIS-C are less likely to experience respiratory symptoms (5–43%), which are the primary signs and symptoms of SARS-CoV-2 infection. These

Clinical features	Percentage (%) according to article									
	Jiang et al. [6]	Santos et al. [7]	Hoste et al. [8]	Radia et al. [9]	Ahmed et al. [10]	Dhar et al. [11]	Kornitzer et al. [12]	Williams et al. [13]	Sood et al. [14]	Miller et al., 2021 [15]
Fever	91	96	97	100	100	100	98	96	85	100
Gastrointestinal involvement[a]	52	46	63	71	74	63	57	86	69	69
Cardiovascular involvement[b]	30	58	32	40	45	23	NR	65	65	78
Shock[c]	38	31	44	61[1]	NR	NR[2]	21	65	40	45
Mucocutaneous involvement[d]	50	38	49	42	56	NR[3]	19	58	52	55
Respiratory symptoms[e]	42	25	31	5	18	NR[4]	14	43	45	29
Neurologic symptoms[f]	27	23	NR	NR	20	16	14	32	26	45
Musculoskeletal symptoms[g]	NR	NR	NR	NR	19	NR	10	17	NR	30
Others[h]	19	NR	NR	NR	13	NR[5]	7	24	NR	22

[a] *(diarrhea, vomiting, abdominal pain, loss of appetite, emesis, poor oral intake).*
[b] *(tachycardia, myocarditis, mild or moderate decreased left ventricular ejection fraction, pericardial effusions).*
[c] *(reported also as a toxic shock, hemodynamic shock, or hypotension).*
[d] *(tongue swelling, erythema and rash, rash, non-purulent conjunctivitis, polymorphous exanthema, erythema and edema of hands and feet, swollen hands and feet, cheilitis).*
[e] *(Cough, dyspnea, shortness of breath, chest tightness, sore throat, rhinorrhea, nasal congestion, pharyngeal erythema).*
[f] *(headache, dizziness, confusion, somnolence, altered mental status, lethargy, fussy, meningeal signs, seizures, sleep disturbance).*
[g] *(extremity findings, myalgia/malaise, edema to extremities).*
[h] *(lymphadenopathy, cervical lymphadenopathy, neck swelling, neck pain fatigue or drowsiness, chest pain, periorbital edema).*
[1] *reported as hypotension.*
[2] *NR (Not reported) reported as most; hypotension.*
[3] *NR (Not reported) reported as some; conjunctivitis, rash, swollen hands and feet.*
[4] *NR (Not reported) reported as most; oxygen requirement, some; cough, sore throat.*
[5] *NR (Not reported) reported as some; lymphadenopathy, neck swelling.*

Table 2.
Clinical features of multisystem inflammatory syndrome in children according to reported study [6–15].

symptoms include cough (5–25%), dyspnea or shortness of breath (11–18%), pharyngeal erythema (32%), lung respiratory distress (11%), rhinorrhea or nasal congestion (7%), sore throat (3%), and chest tightness (2%).

Patients with MIS-C are also less likely to experience meningeal signs, seizures, headache, dizziness, confusion, somnolence, altered mental status, fussiness, or other neurological symptoms (14–32%).

The rarest manifestations of MIS-C patients, although not limited to them, are lymphadenopathy or cervical lymphadenopathy (7–24%), musculoskeletal symptoms or myalgia or malaise (10–30%), and fatigue or drowsiness (9%).

The percentage of reported clinical manifestations in a significant number of MIS-C patients analyzed in this chapter is shown in **Table 2**.

3. Complications of multisystem inflammatory syndrome in children

3.1 Cardiovascular complications of MIS-C

MIS-C represents a severe complication of COVID-19 in children and a potentially life-threatening illness, the severity of which is primarily influenced by the involvement of the cardiovascular system [15].

The most common cardiovascular abnormalities that occur in patients with MIS-C are cardiac dysfunction, particularly left ventricular dysfunction, coronary artery dilation or aneurysm, myocarditis, pericarditis, and congestive heart failure [6–8, 10, 11, 13–15]. Other severe cardiovascular manifestations are hypotension and shock, which are two of the most frequent indications for vasoactive support [6–8, 10, 11, 13–15].

Article	Complications	Number of cases	Percentage %
Jiang et al., [6]	Shock	1146/3036	38
	Myocarditis	830/2829	29
Santos et al., [7]	Shock	675/1544	44
	Hypotension	890/1697	52
Hoste et al., [8]	Hemodynamic shock or hypotension	416/695	56
	Myocarditis	128/309	41
	Mild or moderate decreased LVEF between 30 and 55%;	211/522	40
	LVEF less than 30%	36/506	7
	Coronary dilatation[1]	74/638	12
	Coronary aneurysms[2]	59/572	10
	Pericardial effusion	114/511	22
Ahmed et al., [10]	Shock	398/662	60
	Depressed LVEF	262/662	45
	Depressed LVEF between 30 and 55%	165/662	26
	LVEF less than 30%	33/662	5
	Coronary aneurysms	47/662	8
	Coronary dilatation	50/662	8

Article	Complications	Number of cases	Percentage %
Dhar et al., [11]	Myocarditis	191/309	61
	LVEF (<50%)	190/422	45
	Pericardial involvement[3]	135/436	31
	Coronary artery abnormality	117/681	25
Williams et al., [13]	Shock	363/558	65
	Myocarditis[4]	363/558	65
	LVEF (<55%)[5]	368/603	61
	Coronary artery abnormality	96/248	39
	Coronary artery dilatation	108/681	16
	Coronary artery aneurysm[6]	44/551	8
	Pericardial effusion	166/477	35
Sood et al., [14]	Shock	357/725	49
	Myocarditis	276/870	32
	Left ventricle dysfunction[7]	337/ 823	41
	Coronary vessel abnormalities	143/802	18
	Pericardial effusion	146/709	20
Miller et all., [15]	Shock[8]	2018/4470	45
	Myocarditis	665/4470	15
	Cardiac dysfunction[9]	1296/4198	31
	Pericardial effusion/pericarditis	989/4470	22

LVEF; Left ventricular ejection fraction.[1]*(z-score between 2.0 and 2.5).*
[2]*(z-score above 2.5).*
[3]*Includes asymptomatic, echocardiographic pericardial effusion and pericarditis.*
[4]*(clinical and/or biochemical and/or echocardiography).*
[5]*Myocardial dysfunction or ejection fraction <55%.*
[6]*coronary artery diameter > 2.5 z-score.*
[7]*Abnormal ECHO with left ventricle dysfunction.*
[8]*Receipt of vasopressors.*
[9]*Includes specified left ventricular dysfunction (n = 1151) and right ventricular dysfunction (n = 304); percentages calculated among 4198 persons with an echocardiogram performed.*

Table 3.
Cardiovascular complications of multisystem inflammatory syndrome in children according to reported study [6–8, 10, 11, 13–15].

Cardiac involvement can occur along a spectrum of disease severity in up to 80% of patients with MIS-C [15]. Ventricular dysfunction is a common finding of MIS-C, with up to 61% of patients affected, from the evidence of ventricular function on echocardiography (26–31% of them have mild or moderate decreased of left ventricular ejection fraction-LVEF , whereas less than 10% have severe decreased LVEF) [8, 10, 11, 13, 14].

The evidence of myocarditis, mainly through the clinical picture of myocarditis and elevated cardiac enzymes, is present in up to 65% of children with MIS-C [13]. Myocarditis is one of the main pathophysiological mechanisms of ventricular dysfunction; however, some MIS-C cases have normal levels of cardiac enzymes but depressed ventricular function, suggesting an alternate pathogenesis such as generalized inflammation or changes in loading conditions [17].

Less common cardiovascular complications, but not limited to, are coronary artery abnormalities (18–39%), dilatation (8–16%), or aneurisms (8–10%) [8, 10, 11, 13, 14].

Pericardial involvement, such as pericardial effusion or pericarditis, is also a common complication of MISC (20–35%) [8, 11, 13–15] (**Table 3**).

3.2 Thrombotic events in MIS-C patients

In addition to the hyperinflammatory state, MIS-C is characterized by hypercoagulability and an increased risk of thrombotic events (TEs), particularly in patients with significant ventricular dysfunction or coronary artery aneurysm [18]. Along with elevated inflammatory markers, the majority of patients with MIS-C have elevated serum D-dimer and fibrinogen concentrations, necessitating anticoagulant medication for the majority of them [19].

Pediatric intensive care unit hospitalization, central venous catheterization, cardiac failure, mechanical ventilation, extracorporeal membrane oxygenation, obesity, or other hematological-associated disorders are also risk factors for thromboembolic events in MIS-C patients [18, 19].

The reported incidence of thrombotic events as a complication of MIS-C ranges from 1.4 to 6.5% (**Table 4**) [8, 15, 18, 21, 22].

Thrombotic events in MIS-C patients might be arterial, venous, or intracardiac, with deep vein thrombosis, pulmonary embolism, cerebral artery thrombosis, and thrombotic renal microangiopathy being the most common [15, 24].

Arterial thrombosis can involve as well as coronary arteries, carotid arteries, peripheral systemic arteries, and the aorta. Deep venous thrombosis can affect the deep veins of the lower and upper limbs, the superior vena cava, the internal jugular vein, and the cerebral sinus vein [18, 19, 21, 22]. Intracardiac thrombosis can occur in any of the heart's chambers [18].

The splenic infarctions and hemorrhagic cerebral strokes during extracorporeal membrane oxygenation (ECMO) were also reported as thrombotic complications; however, although abnormal coagulation parameters are frequently reported, thrombotic or embolic events were rare, in contrast to adult COVID-19 [8], but with higher mortality rate [17], as shown in **Table 4**.

3.3 Other severe system involvement in MIS-C patients

Acute kidney injury (AKI) occurs in approximately 12–35% of the patients with MIS-C and is associated with poor prognosis in critically ill children [10, 13, 15, 20]. The incidence of AKI as a complication of MIS-C in a systematic review and meta-analysis with a larger sample size reported by Tripathi et al. is 20% (**Table 4**).

Dehydration, low cardiac output, cytokine storm, the virus's direct cytotoxic action on renal tubular cells, and the use of nephrotoxic medications all can contribute to AKI in MIS-C patients [20]. However, renal hypoperfusion is the main trigger of AKI onset in MIS-C patients [20].

In contrast to the typical pediatric COVID-19 infection, which primarily affects the pulmonary parenchyma and manifests as severe pneumonia, respiratory involvement in children with MIS-C is characterized by pulmonary edema and pleural effusions in the context of multiorgan involvement [25].

Article	Complications	Number of cases	Percentage %
Hoste et al., [8]	Thrombotic complications[1]	13/953	1.4
Miller et al., [15]	Thrombotic complications[2]	38/4470	1
Aronoff et al., [21]	Thrombotic complications[3]	8/229	3.5
Whitworth et al., [22]	Thrombotic complications[4]	9/138	6.5
Maniscalco et al., [18][5]	Thrombotic complications[5]	60	
	Arterial	42/60	70
	Venous	15/60	25
	Intracardiac	14/60	23
Aronoff et al., [21]	AKI	42/353	12
Ahmed et al., [10]	AKI	108/662	16
Bowen et al., [23]	AKI	535/4470	19
Miller et al., [15]	AKI	849/2818	19
Sood et al., [14]	AKI	151/768	20
Tripathi et al., [20]	AKI	990/4947	20
Williams et al., [13]	AKI	166/477	35
Sood et al., [14]	Pleural effusion	101/625	16
	ARDS	40/594	8
Bowen et al., [23]	Pneumonia	747/2818	27
Miller et al., [15]	Pneumonia	1044/4470	23
	Pleural effusion	954 /4470	21
	Acute respiratory distress syndrome	261/4470	6
Miller et al., [15]	Severe hematologic[6]	2663/4470	60
	Severe respiratory[7]	1962/4470	44
	Severe gastrointestinal[8]	1133/4470	25
	Severe renal[9]	908/4470	20
	Severe neurologic[10]	382/4470	9

AKI: Acute kidney injury.
ARDS: Acute respiratory distress syndrome.[1]*Including 2 splenic infarctions, (hemorrhagic) cerebral strokes during extracorporeal membrane oxygenation (ECMO) (n = 5), a recognized complication, contributed substantially to thrombotic complications.*
[2]*Deep vein thrombosis/pulmonary embolism.*
[3]*Deep vein thrombosis and/or pulmonary embolism were identified in 8 of 229 (3.5%).*
[4]*Deep vein thromboses [7], intracardiac thromboses [1], acute ischemic stroke [1].*
[5]*Reports of thrombosis in MIS-C patients published from May 2020 through November 2022.*
[6]*Thrombocytopenia (42%), under signs and symptoms or calculated from laboratory results as platelets; Lymphopenia (35%), lymphocyte count <4500 cells/μl if age < 8 months or < 1500 cells/μl if age ≥ 8 months; Neutropenia (47%), absolute neutrophil count; Deep vein thrombosis/pulmonary embolism (1%).*
[7]*Oxygen, high flow nasal cannula (17%), Invasive mechanical ventilation (intubation) (9%), Non-invasive mechanical ventilation (8%).*
[8]*Free fluid (25%), hepatomegaly/splenomegaly (11%), colitis/enteritis (10%), cholecystitis/gallbladder abnormalities (7%), appendicitis/appendiceal changes (4%).*
[9]*Renal failure (3%) and receipt of dialysis (0.9%).*
[10]*Meningitis (5%), Encephalopathy (4%), Stroke (0.6%).*

Table 4.
Other complications of multisystem inflammatory syndrome in children according to a reported study [8, 10, 13, 15, 20–23].

Severe respiratory involvement, including pneumonia, pleural effusion, and acute respiratory distress syndrome, occurs less frequently 6–27%; however, many MIS-C patients with severe presentation of the disease require any form of respiratory support [15, 23].

Other less prevalent MIS-C complications that have been recorded in a few cases are severe neurological problems 0.6–5% as follows: meningitis, meningoencephalitis, autoimmune encephalitis, encephalopathy, and acute cerebrovascular accidents such as ischemic stroke, intracerebral hemorrhage, subarachnoid hemorrhage, multiple diffuse microhemorrhages, and cerebral sinus venous thrombosis [15, 26].

Reversible splenial lesions, benign intracranial hypertension or pseudotumor cerebri, acute disseminated encephalomyelitis, cranial nerves impairment, transverse myelitis, and fatal cerebral edema have also been reported [26].

Abnormal findings on abdominal imaging, such as free fluid, colitis/enteritis, mesenteric adenitis, hepatomegaly/splenomegaly, gallbladder, and appendix inflammation, are the most prevalent sequelae of severe gastrointestinal involvement 4–25% [15].

4. Sequelae and death causes in MIS-C

The majority of patients with MIS-C had a severe course of the disease that required intensive care unit (ICU) or pediatric intensive care unit (PICU) admission (61–76%), requiring supplemental oxygen via high-flow nasal cannula up to 18%, noninvasive ventilation (8–26%), and invasive mechanical ventilation (9–28%), whereas a small number of cases (4–7%) required ECMO [6–11, 13–15].

A substantial percentage of MIS-C cases, up to 63%, need vasoactive support due to hypotension, shock, and cardiovascular involvement [9].

Short-term morbidity is significant in terms of requiring intensive care treatments; MIS-C patients frequently require special care and vigorous treatment. Nonetheless, the majority of patients have favorable outcomes, and overall mortality is low (0.8%–2.41%), as shown in **Table 5**.

Children who have one or more underlying medical conditions, the most prevalent of which is obesity, have a higher mortality rate [23].

Mortality is higher among children who have had a longer duration of the disease prior to being admitted to the PICU, have severe involvement of four to five organ systems, more cardiovascular complications and shock, severe involvement of the respiratory system, and require more mechanical ventilation support and renal replacement therapy [23, 27, 28].

Furthermore, non-survivor patients have more neurological or respiratory symptoms, less diarrhea, and normal nutritional status; they also have higher levels of blood D-dimer, ferritin, lactate, and CRP [27, 28].

Most patients with MIS-C have good outcomes with no significant sequelae one year after diagnosis [3]. Laboratory abnormalities including NTproBNP, troponin-T, lymphocytopenia, thrombocytopenia, and C-reactive protein (CRP), normalize within 1–4 weeks after hospitalization [29].

Almost all cardiac abnormalities, including serum biomarkers and ventricular dysfunction (LV systolic dysfunction, LV ejection fraction, and LV systolic dysfunction), recover within 6 weeks to 6 months of follow-up; however, coronary artery abnormalities in a small percentage of MIS-C patients persist but improve after 6 months [29, 30].

Author		Number of MIS-C cases	Percentage %
Jiang et al., [6] Number of MIS-C cases; 4475	ICU	2050/3163	65
	MV	666/3901	17
	ECMO	64/2654	2
	Inotropes	971/2565	38
	Deaths	76/3159	2.41
Santos et al., [7] Number of MIS-C cases; 2144	ICU	1294/1973	66
	(MV/NIV/ HFNC)	731/1919	38
	ECMO	36/641	7
	Inotropes	313/1965	16
	Death	38/1973	2
Hoste et al., [8] Number of MIS-C cases; 953	ICU	564/769	73
	MV	219/928	24
	NIV	130/503	26
	ECMO	36/953	4
	Severe course[1]	118/138	86
	Inotropes	477/863	55
Radia et al., [9] Number of MIS-C cases; 783	ICU	531/783	68
	MV	138/783	18
	NIV	87/783	11
	HFNC	22/783	3
	ECMO	31/783	4
	Inotropes	436/688	63
	Deaths	12/783	1.5
Ahmed et al., [10] Number of MIS-C cases; 662	ICU	469/662	71
	MV	147/662	22
	ECMO	29/662	4
	Inotropes	347/662	52
	Deaths	11/662	1·7
Dhar et al., [11] Number of MIS-C cases; 883	Inotropes	458/783	61
	MV	226/813	28
	Deaths	13/833	1·6%
Williams et al., [13]	PICU[c]	633/833	76
	MV	208/833	25
	NIV	109/497	22
	HFNC	70/389	18
	ECMO	33/833	4
	Inotropes	508/833	61
	Deaths	18/833	2.1

Author		Number of MIS-C cases	Percentage %
Sood et al., [14] Number of MIS-C cases; 992	ICU	551/872	63
	MV	183/872	21
	Inotropes	363/872	42
	Deaths	22/992	2.2
Miller et al., [15] Reported MIS-C case; 4470	ICU	2793/4470	63
	MV	419/4470	9
	NIV	368/4470	8
	HFNC	753/4470	17
	Inotropes	2018/4470	45
	Deaths	35/4470	0.8%

Abbreviations: PICU/ICU, pediatric intensive care unit; MV; mechanical ventilation; NIV; noninvasive ventilation; HFNC, high-flow nasal cannula; ECMO, extracorporeal membrane oxygenation.[1]Severe course was defined as the presence of coronary dilatation/aneurysm, shock, death, need for mechanical ventilation, extracorporeal membrane oxygenation (ECMO), renal replacement therapy, inotropes, or PICU admission.

Table 5.
Outcomes of multisystem inflammatory syndrome in children according to reported study [6–11, 13–15].

Furthermore, most organ-specific complications resolve by 6 months post-diagnosis; complications persisting at 6 months include muscular fatigue, abnormalities at neurological examination, anxiety, and emotional difficulties [3].

Patients with MIS-C treated with immunomodulators have favorable early outcomes with no mortality, normalization of LV systolic function, recovery of coronary abnormalities, and no inflammation or scarring on cardiac MRI [31].

5. Conclusion

MIS-C is a severe complication of the SARS-CoV-2 infection that generally appears 2–6 weeks after infection and is common in previously healthy children; most of them manifest asymptomatic or mild forms of the COVID-19 infection, and it seems to develop in the post-infectious stage rather than during the acute infection stage of COVID-19.

MIS-C can occur at any age in children, but it is more common in children aged 7–9 years and more frequent in boys and in children with obesity.

The symptom complex of fever, GI symptoms, cardiac involvement, and rash or KD-like symptoms in children with prior symptomatic or asymptomatic SARS-CoV-2 infection, should prompt clinicians to recognize this syndrome early.

The involvement of the cardiovascular system and thromboembolic problems, which are the most prevalent sequelae of MIS-C, have the largest influence on the severity of this illness.

Short-term morbidity is significant in terms of requiring intensive care and vigorous treatment; nonetheless, the majority of patients have favorable outcomes, with no significant sequelae one year after diagnosis, and overall mortality is low.

Acronyms and abbreviations

AKI	acute kidney injury
ECMO	extracorporeal membrane oxygenation
ICU	intensive care unit
LVEF	left ventricular ejection fraction
MIS-C	multisystem inflammatory syndrome in children
PTT	partial thromboplastin time
PICU	pediatric intensive care unit
PT	prothrombin time
SARS-CoV-2	severe acute respiratory syndrome coronavirus 2
TEs	thrombotic events

Author details

Alije Keka-Sylaj
Institute of Anatomy, Faculty of Medicine, University of Prishtina, Pediatric Clinic, University Clinical Center of Kosovo, Prishtina, Kosovo

*Address all correspondence to: alije.keka@uni-pr.edu

References

[1] Riphagen S, Gomez X, Gonzalez-Martinez C, Wilkinson N, Theocharis P. Hyperinflammatory shock in children during COVID-19 pandemic. Lancet. 2020;**395**(10237):1607-1608

[2] Keka-Sylaj A, Ramosaj A, Baloku A, Zogaj L, Gjaka P. Multisystem inflammatory syndrome in children (MIS-C), possibly due to COVID-19 mRNA vaccination. Vaccines (Basel). 2023;**11**(5):956

[3] CDC. Centers for Disease Control and Prevention. 2020 [cited 2023 Apr 22]. Multisystem Inflammatory Syndrome (MIS). Available from: https://www.cdc.gov/mis/mis-c/hcp_cstecdc/index.html

[4] Multisystem Inflammatory Syndrome in Children and Adolescents Temporally Related to COVID-19 [Internet]. [cited 2023 Aug 6]. Available from: https://www.who.int/news-room/commentaries/detail/multisystem-inflammatory-syndrome-in-children-and-adolescents-with-covid-19

[5] Esposito S, Principi N. Multisystem Inflammatory Syndrome in Children Related to SARS-CoV-2. Pediatric Drugs. Mar 2021;**23**(2):119-129

[6] Jiang L, Tang K, Irfan O, Li X, Zhang E, Bhutta Z. Epidemiology, clinical features, and outcomes of multisystem inflammatory syndrome in children (MIS-C) and adolescents-a live systematic review and meta-analysis. Current Pediatrics Reports. 2022;**10**(2):19-30

[7] Santos MO, Gonçalves LC, Silva PAN, Moreira ALE, Ito CRM, Peixoto FAO, et al. Multisystem inflammatory syndrome (MIS-C): A systematic review and meta-analysis of clinical characteristics, treatment, and outcomes. Jornal de Pediatria. 2021;**98**(4):338-349

[8] Hoste L, Van Paemel R, Haerynck F. Multisystem inflammatory syndrome in children related to COVID-19: A systematic review. European Journal of Pediatrics. 2021;**180**(7):2019-2034

[9] Radia T, Williams N, Agrawal P, Harman K, Weale J, Cook J, et al. Multi-system inflammatory syndrome in children & adolescents (MIS-C): A systematic review of clinical features and presentation. Paediatric Respiratory Reviews. 2021;**38**:51-57

[10] Ahmed M, Advani S, Moreira A, Zoretic S, Martinez J, Chorath K, et al. Multisystem inflammatory syndrome in children: A systematic review. EClinicalMedicine. 2020;**26**:100527

[11] Dhar D, Dey T, Samim MM, Padmanabha H, Chatterjee A, Naznin P, et al. Systemic inflammatory syndrome in COVID-19–SISCoV study: Systematic review and meta-analysis. Pediatric Research. 2022;**91**(6):1334-1349

[12] Kornitzer J, Johnson J, Yang M, Pecor KW, Cohen N, Jiang C, et al. A systematic review of characteristics associated with COVID-19 in children with typical presentation and with multisystem inflammatory syndrome. International Journal of Environmental Research and Public Health. 2021;**18**(16):8269

[13] Williams V, Dash N, Suthar R, Mohandoss V, Jaiswal N, Kavitha TK, et al. Clinicolaboratory profile, treatment, intensive care needs, and outcome of Pediatric inflammatory multisystem syndrome temporally associated with SARS-CoV-2: A systematic review and

meta-analysis. Journal of Pediatric Intensive Care. 2020;**11**(1):1-12

[14] Sood M, Sharma S, Sood I, Sharma K, Kaushik A. Emerging evidence on multisystem inflammatory syndrome in children associated with SARS-CoV-2 infection: A systematic review with meta-analysis. SN Comprehensive Clinical Medicine. 2021;**3**(1):38-47

[15] Miller AD, Zambrano LD, Yousaf AR, Abrams JY, Meng L, Wu MJ, et al. MIS-C Surveillance Authorship Group. Multisystem inflammatory syndrome in children—United States, February 2020–July 2021. Clinical Infectious Diseases. 24 Aug 2022;**75**(1):e1165-e1175

[16] Alkan G, Sert A, Oz SKT, Emiroglu M, Yılmaz R. Clinical features and outcome of MIS-C patients: An experience from Central Anatolia. Clinical Rheumatology. 2021;**40**(10):4179-4189

[17] Wu EY, Campbell MJ. Cardiac manifestations of multisystem inflammatory syndrome in children (MIS-C) following COVID-19. Current Cardiology Reports. 2021;**23**(11):168

[18] Maniscalco V, Niccolai R, Marrani E, Maccora I, Bertini F, Pagnini I, et al. Thrombotic events in MIS-C patients: A single case report and literature review. Children. 2023;**10**(4):618

[19] Kumar R, Rivkin MJ, Raffini L. Thrombotic complications in children with Coronavirus disease 2019 and Multisystem Inflammatory Syndrome of Childhood. Journal of Thrombosis and Haemostasis. Sep 2023;**21**(9):2313-2326

[20] Tripathi AK, Pilania RK, Bhatt GC, Atlani M, Kumar A, Malik S. Acute kidney injury following multisystem inflammatory syndrome associated with SARS-CoV-2 infection in children: A systematic review and meta-analysis. Pediatric Nephrology. 2023;**38**(2):357-370

[21] Aronoff SC, Hall A, Del Vecchio MT. The natural history of severe acute respiratory syndrome coronavirus 2–related multisystem inflammatory syndrome in children: A systematic review. Journal of the Pediatric Infectious Diseases Society. 2020;**9**(6):746-751

[22] Whitworth H, Sartain SE, Kumar R, Armstrong K, Ballester L, Betensky M, et al. Rate of thrombosis in children and adolescents hospitalized with COVID-19 or MIS-C. Blood. 2021;**138**(2):190-198

[23] Bowen A, Miller AD, Zambrano LD, Wu MJ, Oster ME, Godfred-Cato S, et al. Demographic and clinical factors associated with death among persons <21 years old with multisystem inflammatory syndrome in children—United States, February 2020–march 2021. Open Forum Infectious Diseases. 2021;**8**(8):ofab388

[24] Bregel LV, Efremova OS, Kostyunin KY, Rudenko NY, Kozlov YA, Albot VV, et al. Thrombosis in multisystem inflammatory syndrome associated with COVID-19 in children: Retrospective cohort study analysis and review of the literature. Biomedicine. 2023;**11**(8):2206

[25] Winant AJ, Blumfield E, Liszewski MC, Kurian J, Foust AM, Lee EY. Thoracic imaging findings of multisystem inflammatory syndrome in children associated with COVID-19: What radiologists need to know now. Radiology: Cardiothoracic Imaging. 2020;**2**(4):e200346

[26] Siracusa L, Cascio A, Giordano S, Medaglia AA, Restivo GA, Pirrone I, et al. Neurological complications in pediatric patients with SARS-CoV-2 infection:

A systematic review of the literature. Italian Journal of Pediatrics. 2021;**47**:123

[27] Acevedo L, Piñeres-Olave BE, Niño-Serna LF, Vega LM, Gomez IJA, Chacón S, et al. Mortality and clinical characteristics of multisystem inflammatory syndrome in children (MIS-C) associated with covid-19 in critically ill patients: An observational multicenter study (MISCO study). BMC Pediatrics. 2021;**21**(1):516

[28] Sık G, Inamlık A, Akçay N, Kesici S, Aygun F, Kendırlı T, et al. Mortality risk factors among critically ill children with MIS-C in PICUs: A multicenter study. Pediatric Research. 2023;**94**(2):730-737

[29] Fremed MA, Farooqi KM. Longitudinal outcomes and monitoring of patients with multisystem inflammatory syndrome in children. Frontiers in Pediatrics. 1 Apr 2022;**10**:820229

[30] Yasuhara J, Masuda K, Watanabe K, Shirasu T, Takagi H, Sumitomo N, et al. Longitudinal cardiac outcomes of multisystem inflammatory syndrome in children: A systematic review and meta-analysis. Pediatric Cardiology. 2023;**44**(4):892-907

[31] Capone CA, Misra N, Ganigara M, Epstein S, Rajan S, Acharya SS, et al. Six month follow-up of patients with multi-system inflammatory syndrome in children. Pediatrics. 2021;**148**(4):e2021050973